Seniors Choosing to Prolong Living
Technologies and Ethics for Life Extension
Mark Roberts-Seymour, PEng, OFS

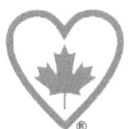

Seniors Life Extension

Published by Secular Orders Press
Vernon, BC, Canada V1T 9W3
1018 – 4900 – 20th Street

Library of Congress Cataloguing:
Mark E. Roberts-Seymour, OFS (1948-)
~~Life Extension for Seniors Book 1: Expectations, Ageing Inhibition, Nutrition, Brain 'Wiring', Habits, Exercise and Ethics~~ Seniors Choosing to Prolong Living
Technologies and Ethics for Life Extension
1. Biology of Ageing, 2. Brain-Mind, 3. Title

ISBN 9781718128514 ~~978-1-989037-19-5~~
Copyright © 2018 by Mark Roberts-Seymour
All Rights Reserved

Seniors Life Extension

Life Extension for Seniors
Book 1
Expectations, Ageing Inhibition, Nutrition, Brain 'Wiring', Habits, Exercise and Ethics

Mark Roberts-Seymour, PEng.

Seniors Life Extension

Introduction

This book presents foundation keys, rationalisations and outlines techniques for the extension of life. It is intended to be read by those at their age of impending 'retirement' and those already retired. One of the most socially critical problems facing North Americans today is that their jobs, satisfaction from accomplishment and any hope of a sound financial base are fast disappearing as machine technology causes 'redundancy' in the workplace. Many workers are faced with earlier and earlier ages of retirement. In most cases this is not their choice, but spirited efforts to get re-employed are met with poor prospects, and while they are technically *'discouraged workers',* they become to all practical purposes 'retired'. There is controversy as to what the new age of retirement is [or ought to be], since the capacity to work goes well beyond age 65, while the prospects to stay in a conventional wage-role beyond age 50 are dimming. With exceptions, individuals are living longer and longer lives – and want to do so. Getting and staying 'healthy' is essential to life extension. What you do with the extension is a separate issue – a circumstance that you alone can manage.

Currently the most significant population trend is ageing, with 11% of the world's current population aged 60 and older. The United Nations Population Fund (UNFPA) estimates that by 2050 that number will rise to approximately 22%. Ageing of populations appears tied to five global improvements:

1. nutrition,
2. sanitation,

3. health care,
4. education and
5. economic well-being.

None of these five are expected to retreat globally, and improvements especially in developing nations are progressing rapidly. Fertility rates have continued to decline and life expectancy has risen. As life expectancy rises and birth rates decline in developed countries, the median age rises accordingly. According to the United Nations, this process is taking place in nearly every country in the world. A rising median age can have significant social and economic implications, as the workforce gets progressively older and the number of old workers and retirees grows relative to the number of young workers. Older people generally incur more health-related costs than do younger people in the workplace and can also cost more in worker's compensation and pension liabilities. In most developed countries an older workforce appears inevitable, though the influence of the 'machine workforces' still is neither quantified or adequately anticipated.

Income Security

Among the most urgent concerns of older persons worldwide is income security. This poses challenges for governments with ageing populations to ensure investment in pension systems continues in order to provide economic independence and reduce poverty in old age. All these systems take from the employed [the younger working members of the society] - and allocate them either by direct payments to the retired person or through income from tangible investments made from such contributions in the economy of the nation. In both instances the balance or ratio between those paying into the system and those taking out [the pensioners] is delicate. If projections are correct, within thirty years the takers will have doubled in number while the contributors will have dwindled. A 'crisis' is a mild term for the future of developed nation pension schemes. Either pensions will decrease proportional to the number of pensioners, or contributions will have to rise to accommodate the increased payout pressure dictated by the number of pensions offered. These challenges vary for developing and developed countries. UNFPA stated recently: "Sustainability of these systems is of particular concern, particularly in developed countries - while social protection and old-age pension coverage remain a challenge for developing countries, where a large proportion of the labour force is found in the *informal sector.*"

Due to increasing share of the elderly in the population, health care expenditures will continue to grow relative to the economy in coming decades. This has been considered as a negative phenomenon and effective strategies like labour productivity enhancement should be considered to deal with negative consequences of ageing.

Seniors Life Extension

Life Expectancy

While it contains one of a number of basic flaws the Life Expectancy at Birth (LEB) is the most common measure of how many years we will live. These figures do include infant mortality (in the first six years of life) which skews the numbers considerably as we will see. If you reach 50 years of age, your remaining life is anticipated to exceed the LEB from your birth year. The 2017 LEB for Canadian Males was 79 years and for Canadian Females 84 years. It is shorter in the United States, owing in part to their health care delivery system. The gap between the two genders is decreasing (though not as quickly in recent years). Many other factors influence life expectancy: notably where you were born, where you reside, income, education and health.

A Brief History of Life Expectancy

A perspective on the Life Expectancy at Birth historically provides an insight into how rapidly life expectancy began to change. Until after 1950 LEB held to levels of approximately 40% of current levels from the Paleolithic age until 1950 when it began a heady upward spiral. Health care improvements together with access to it, lack of large-scale warfare, agricultural improvements and improved working conditions have all contributed to the increase. In recent years this increase trend has slowed, but life expectancy is still escalating.

From 1950 to 2014 the world life expectancy jumped by fifty percent. Projections vary considerably: but before 2050 it is quite likely to exceed 100 years (it already does for those now living to age 90, if in good health). The following Table indicates some benchmark life spans divided by era:

Era	Life expectancy at birth in years	Threshold % of Canadian 2017 LEB
Paleolithic	33	
Neolithic	20 to 33	41.3
Bronze Age and Iron Age	26	
Classical Greece	25 to 28	35.0
Classical Rome	20–30	37.5
Pre-Columbian Southern United States	25–30	37.5
Medieval Islamic Caliphate[	35+	
Late medieval English peerage	30	
Early modern England	33–40	50.0
Pre-Champlain Canadian Maritimes	60	75.0
18th-century Prussia	24.7	30.9
18th-century France	27.5–30	37.5
18th-century Qing	39.6	49.5

Era	Life expectancy at birth in years	Threshold % of Canadian 2017 LEB
China		
18th-century Edo Japan	41.1	
Early 19th-century England	40	51.4
1900 world average	31	38.8
1950 world average	48	60.0
2014 world average	71.5	89.4

Indigenous residents of different countries around the world have different life expectancies; with shortest times in Africa and greatest in highly industrial nations (not withstanding air and water pollutants). The following world map reflects the disparities:

Life expectancy at birth takes account of infant mortality but not prenatal mortality.

Seniors Life Extension

Changes in Life Expectancy: Recent Change

The period from the End of the Spanish Flu (1921) to the most recent data is often cited for life expectancy comparison purposes. In Canada through 2005 a rise of 34.5% among men is shown, while for women the increase was 38%The following table tracks the Canadian experience over those years:

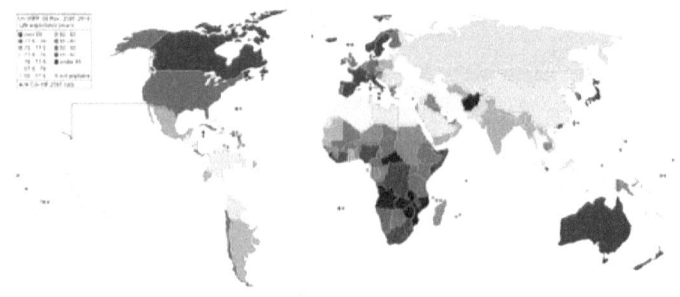

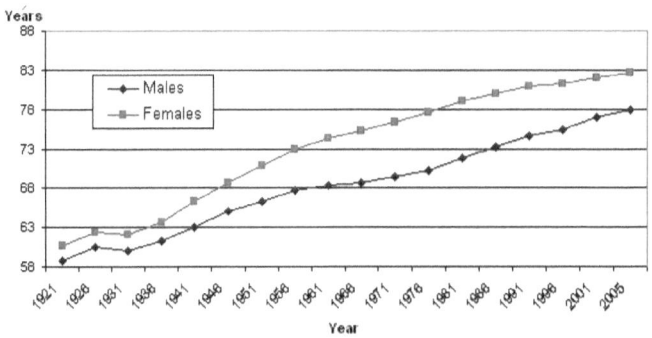

Life expectancy at birth, by sex, Canada, 1956 to 2005

Source: 1921 to 1981: Nagnur D. *Longevity and Historical Life Tables, 1921 to 1981 (Abridged)*, Statistics Canada, Catalogue 98-506, 1986;
1986: Duchesne D, Nault F, Gilmour H, Wilkins R. *Vital Statistics Compendium 1996*, Statistics Canada, Catalogue 84-214, 1999;
1991 to 2005: CANSIM Table 102-0511, Life expectancy, abridged life table, at birth and at age 65, by sex, Canada, provinces and territories, annual.

Life after Fifty

Individuals living longer 'beat-the-odds' when it comes to life expectancy. Without considering issues of suitable environment, health status and financial security - the following Chart reflects projected remaining life for people as they arrive at benchmark ages:

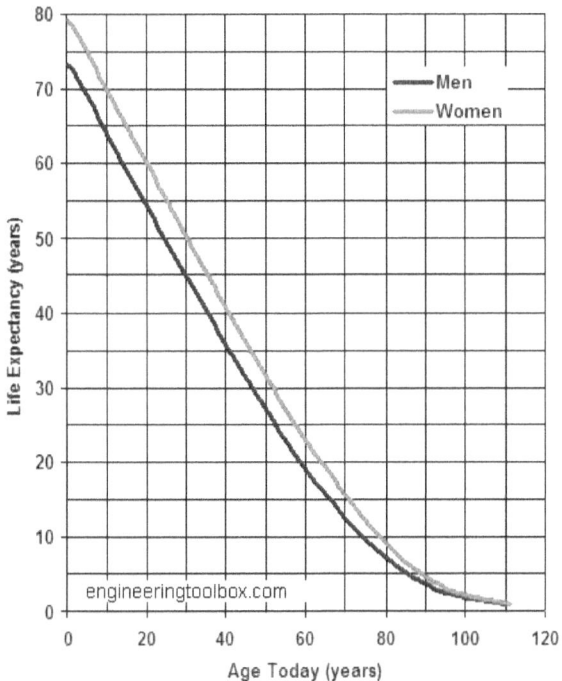

A second chart, using independent data, makes the same case for those surviving longer:

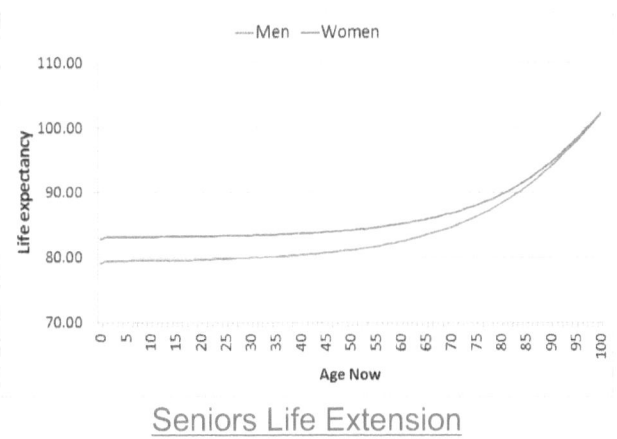

Seniors Life Extension

An approach which relates remaining life to percentiles and average for men 70 and older is as follows:

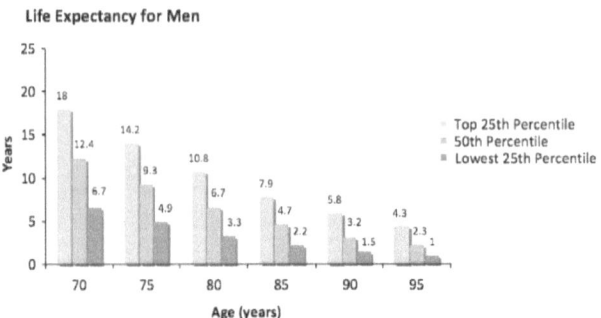

At seventy the remaining year projection is almost 200% higher from the lower quartile to the highest and at 90 is almost 300%. Getting into the highest quartile by working at it will extend life significantly/

Physical Health, Obesity and Life Expectancy

It has become a fact that Obesity is endemic in Industrialized nations and has been, while not as rapidly, is increasing there without abatement. Obesity has been linked to increase of risk of numerous health problems, including high blood pressure, stroke, type 2 diabetes and heart disease. The outcome of these in many cases is premature death. Life span is accordingly reduced when this factor is considered.

In a recent (2013) study overweight was defined as a body mass index (BMI) of 25 kg/m² or higher and obese was defined as a BMI of 30 kg/m² or higher. The researchers found that over the past 33 years, worldwide overweight and obesity rates among adults have increased by 27.5%, while such rates among children and adolescents have increased by 47.1%. Collectively, the number of overweight and obese people worldwide has increased from 857 million in 1980 to 2.1 billion in 2013 – 30% of the world's population. Of these, 671 million or approximately 10% are obese.

Greatest increases in overweight and obesity rates occurred between 1992 and 2002. At present, more than half of the obese worldwide population reside in only 10 countries, including the US, China, Russia, Brazil, Mexico, Egypt, Germany, Pakistan and Indonesia.

62% of the world's obese individuals live in developed countries. The US had the highest increases in prevalence of adult obesity – a third of the population are now obese. This is followed by Australia – where 28% of men and 30% of women are obese – and the UK – where around a quarter of the adult population are obese. More than 50% of women are obese in Kuwait, Libya, Qatar, the Pacific Islands of Kiribati, Federated States of Micronesia and Samoa. Unlike other major global health risks, such as smoking, obesity rates are not falling. The following chart indicates that life span decrease is directly linked to obesity:

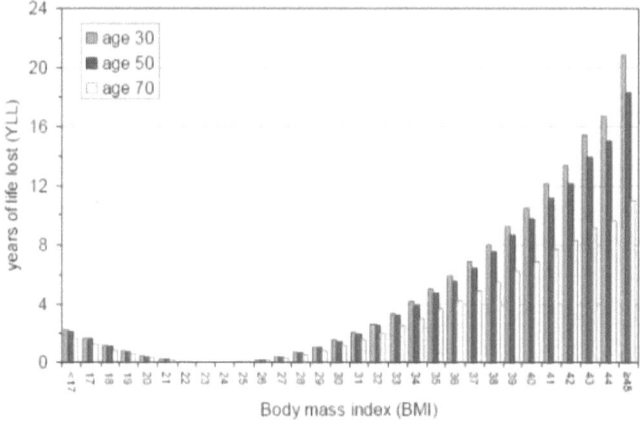

At the bottom threshold of obesity (30 kg/m²), a 50-year-old is shaving more than 2 years off of his/her life expectancy, while the same person if morbidly obese (40kg/m²) sees 11 years lost from his/her lifetime.

Income and Life Expectancy

The Gross Domestic Product per capita is the most influential determinant of life expectancy, with the curve becoming less pronounced above $30000 per capita based on the following graph.

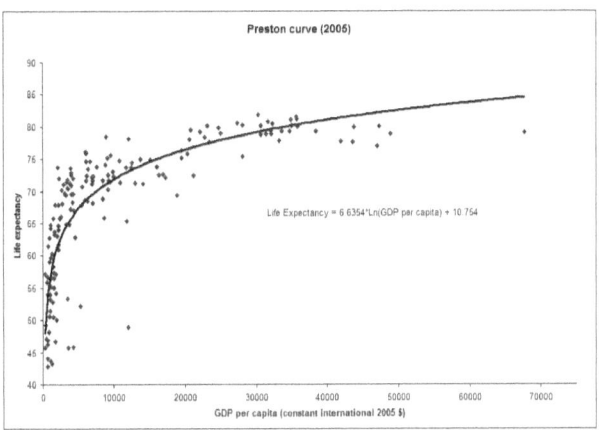

From Highest GDP per capita to lowest it can be seen that the first 34 nations fall above the 30k benchmark:

Rank	Country	GDP – PER CAPITA (PPP)	Date of Information
1	Liechtenstein	$139,100	2009 est.
2	Qatar	$124,900	2017 est.
3	Monaco	$115,700	2015 est.
4	Macau	$114,400	2017 est.
5	Luxembourg	$109,100	2017 est.
6	Falkland Islands (Islas Malvinas)	$96,200	2012 est.
7	Singapore	$90,500	2017 est.
8	Bermuda	$85,700	2013 est.
9	Isle of Man	$84,600	2014 est.
10	Brunei	$76,700	2017 est.
11	Ireland	$72,600	2017 est.
12	Norway	$70,600	2017 est.
13	Kuwait	$69,700	2017 est.
14	United Arab Emirates	$68,200	2017 est.

15	Sint Maarten	$66,800	2014 est.
16	Gibraltar	$61,700	2014 est.
17	Switzerland	$61,400	2017 est.
18	Hong Kong	$61,000	2017 est.
19	San Marino	$59,500	2017 est.
20	United States	$59,500	2017 est.
21	Saudi Arabia	$55,300	2017 est.
22	Netherlands	$53,600	2017 est.
23	Guernsey	$52,500	2014 est.
24	Iceland	$52,100	2017 est.
25	Bahrain	$51,800	2017 est.
26	Sweden	$51,300	2017 est.
27	Germany	$50,200	2017 est.
28	Australia	$49,900	2017 est.
29	Andorra	$49,900	2015 est.
30	Taiwan	$49,800	2017 est.
31	Denmark	$49,600	2017 est.
32	Jersey	$49,500	2015 est.
33	Austria	$49,200	2017 est.
34	Canada	$48,100	2017 est.
35	Belgium	$46,300	2017 est.
36	Oman	$45,500	2017 est.
37	Finland	$44,000	2017 est.
38	Cayman Islands	$43,800	2004 est.
39	France	$43,600	2017 est.
40	United Kingdom	$43,600	2017 est.
41	Japan	$42,700	2017 est.

Seniors Life Extension

42	Malta	$42,500	2017 est.
43	British Virgin Islands	$42,300	2010 est.
44	Faroe Islands	$40,000	2014 est.
45	Korea, South	$39,400	2017 est.
46	European Union	$39,200	2017 est.
47	New Zealand	$38,500	2017 est.
48	Spain	$38,200	2017 est.
49	Italy	$38,000	2017 est.
50	Puerto Rico	$37,900	2017 est.
51	Greenland	$37,600	2015 est.
52	Cyprus	$36,600	2017 est.
53	Israel	$36,200	2017 est.
54	Virgin Islands	$36,100	2013 est.
55	Czechia	$35,200	2017 est.
56	Equatorial Guinea	$34,900	2017 est.
57	Saint Pierre and Miquelon	$34,900	2006 est.
58	Slovenia	$34,100	2017 est.
59	Slovakia	$32,900	2017 est.
60	Lithuania	$31,900	2017 est.
61	Estonia	$31,500	2017 est.
62	Trinidad and Tobago	$31,200	2017 est.
63	New Caledonia	$31,100	2015 est.
64	Guam	$30,500	2013 est.
65	Portugal	$30,300	2017 est.
66	Poland	$29,300	2017 est.

67	Turks and Caicos Islands	$29,100	2007 est.
68	Seychelles	$28,900	2017 est.
69	Hungary	$28,900	2017 est.
70	Malaysia	$28,900	2017 est.
71	Russia	$27,900	2017 est.
72	Greece	$27,800	2017 est.
73	Latvia	$27,300	2017 est.
74	Saint Kitts and Nevis	$26,800	2017 est.
75	Turkey	$26,500	2017 est.
76	Antigua and Barbuda	$26,300	2017 est.
77	Kazakhstan	$26,100	2017 est.
78	Aruba	$25,300	2011 est.
79	Bahamas, The	$25,100	2017 est.
80	Chile	$24,600	2017 est.
81	Panama	$24,300	2017 est.
82	Croatia	$24,100	2017 est.
83	Romania	$24,000	2017 est.

Source CIA Worldbook 2016

Variations within Nation-States

The measured GDP per capita in 2017 (Statscan) was $56,129, significantly raising the ranking in the Worldbook table shown above.

Even within nations the GDP pc varies considerably. In Canada this is represented by the table following:

Seniors Life Extension

GDP PerCapita Canadian Provinces and Territories 2017

Province	GDPpc	Gross GDP	% GDP
Northwest Territories	106,215	4,739	0.23
Alberta	74,343	314,944	15.47
Yukon	73,518	na	0.14
Nunavut	65,713	2,443	0.12
Saskatchewan	65,525	75,261	3.7
Newfoundland and Labrador	58,668	31,112	1.53
Ontario	56,870	794,835	39.05
	55,428	263,706	12.96

British Columbia			
Manitoba	51,485	67,863	3.33
Quebec	47,443	394,819	19.4
New Brunswick	45,187	34,224	1.68
Nova Scotia	43,986	41,726	2.05
Prince Edward Island	42,289	6,321	0.31

Anti-Ageing Traditions

Anti-ageing medicine as a discipline is less than forty years old, at least the jargon that the movement employs is only that old. Indefinite life extension, experimental gerontology, and biomedical gerontology are terms for a study of slowing down or reversing the processes of aging to extend both the maximum and average lifespan. The ability to achieve this, however, does not currently exist. It is the holy grail of this movement, but the results of steps engineered in the last forty years have succeeded in pushing the ageing-envelope or threshold and warrant examination.

Some researchers in this area, and "longevists" (those who wish to achieve longer lives themselves), believe that soon to be realized advances in eight fields of medicine will be critical to their aims:

1. tissue rejuvenation,
2. stem cells,
3. regenerative medicine,
4. molecular repair,
5. gene therapy,
6. Pharmaceuticals and diet maanagement
7. organ replacement
8. artificial organs or xenotransplantations

These do not function severally or in isolation one from another. What works in one potentiates advances in another, and in fact bears on all of the seven others simultaneously. Proponents contend that these technologies, when advanced and integrated, will eventually enable humans to have indefinite lifespans (agerasia) through complete rejuvenation to a healthy youthful condition. There are many ethical ramifications, as life extension becomes more 'probable'. These are currently hotly debated by a cadre of bioethicists, who work with arcane philosophical tools and a paucity of statistical proofs for the most part.

It's Big Business

Marketing alleged 'anti-ageing products' has become lucrative; and is now a self-preserving global aggregate of business dynasties. Their level of self-defense of many wide-spread untruths based on flimsy science and anecdotal 'evidence' often has prevented reasonable advances from being implemented. The profit-margin, not the benefit, drives these corporations. As an example, the industry that promotes the use of hormones as a treatment for consumers to slow or reverse the ageing process self-reported a six billion US dollar sales in 2015. Market strategists estimate a growth rate of 2.5% compounding annually. Other reports place this therapy's sales at more than 50 billion dollars in the United States alone. The use of such products has not been proven to be effective or even safe; but may account for more than $40 per year for every living US adult, and still be advancing. In comparison, the sales of Multi-Vitamins in the US only netted 39 billion dollars in the same period, actually less than the higher threshold estimate for Hormone Replacement Therapeutics alone.

Ageing Mechanics

Before delving deeply into life-extending technology as a matter to debate, consideration must be given to where we have come from. Consider the table included earlier that set out the rise of life expectancy at birth from an historical framework. Man has seen life expectancy more than double since roughly 1540 AD. Now, contrast that with the stated goal of many life-extenders to double [again] the life of man through prolongation technologies. The first set of technologies which resulted in an LEB jump from 30 years to 80 years included; sanitation, nutrition, education and medicine. All arguments positioned here which belittle life-extension research and development could also have been levelled against the first wave of 'enhancement technologies' These brought life expectancy to levels seen today, but nowhere have we a demonstrated historical ethics model which railed against polio vaccine as 'un-natural' and rife with ethical dilemmas.

What is the Strategy for Life-Extension

Ageing is focal to the non-machine life prolongation research and development proposed by life-enhancement adherents. The effort is currently aimed at seven main categories of 'damage' related to ageing, leading to seeking alterations for each. Reversal would constitute negligible senescence:

1. cell loss or atrophy (without replacement),
2. oncogenic nuclear mutations and epimutations,
3. cell senescence (Death-resistant cells),
4. mitochondrial mutations,
5. Intracellular junk or junk inside cells (lysosomal aggregates)
6. extracellular junk or junk outside cells (extracellular aggregates)
7. random extracellular cross-linking

Ageing represents the accumulation of changes in a human being over time, encompassing physical, psychological, and social changes. Reaction time, for example, may slow with age, while knowledge of world events and incipient 'wisdom' likely increases. Ageing is the greatest known risk factors for most human diseases. About two thirds of all persons who die every day do so from age-related causes.

The causes of ageing are uncertain. Accepted current theories are assigned to the damage concept, whereby the accumulation of damage (such as DNA oxidation) may cause biological systems to fail, or to the programmed ageing concept, whereby internal processes (such as DNA methylation) may cause ageing. Programmed ageing should not be confused with programmed cell death (apoptosis).

The ageing process is now considered to reflect ten 'patterns' as an individual accumulates damage to macromolecules, cells, tissues, and organs. Specifically, it is 'influenced' by combinations of:

1. genomic instability, a high frequency of mutations within the genome of a cellular lineage. These mutations can include changes in nucleic acid sequences, chromosomal rearrangements or aneuploidy.

2. telomere attrition, wherein telomeres which allow cells to divide without losing genes are reduced and chromosome ends can fuse together corrupting the cell's genetic blueprint, possibly causing malfunction, cancer, or cell death.

3. epigenetic alterations, heritable alterations that are not due to changes in DNA sequence. Rather, epigenetic modifications, or "tags," such as DNA methylation and histone modification, which alter DNA accessibility and chromatin structure, thereby regulating patterns of gene expression, and may corrupt such presentation in ageing.

4. loss of proteostasis, a loss of protein homeostasis (proteostasis) characterized by the appearance of non-native protein aggregates within tissues. Protein aggregation is routinely suppressed by the proteostasis network (PN), a collection of macromolecular machines that operate in diverse ways to maintain proteome integrity across subcellular compartments and between tissues to ensure a healthy life span, but the loss of which contributes to cellular degradation.

5. deregulated nutrient sensing, wherein a disruption of essential nutrient sensing starting with receptors in the mouth, impede the quality pf sense of taste employed make the decision to ingest calorie-rich food and reject potential toxins and spoiled food. Following ingestion, the contents of the gastrointestinal tract continue to be monitored for their chemical content by the sensing system which may be compromised. Effects include disease processes such as diabetes and obesity.

6. mitochondrial dysfunction, wherein the organelles that generate energy for the cell become dysfunctional, and as constituents of every cell of the human body [except red blood cells], fail to 'correctly' convert the energy of food molecules into the adenosine triphosphate [ATP] that powers most cell functions, leading to unhealthy outcomes.

7. cellular senescence or cellular ageing-degradation, is most commonly triggered by a DNA damage-response resulting from the shortening of telomeres during each cellular division process. Cells can also be induced to senesce independent of the number of cellular divisions via DNA damage in response to elevated reactive oxygen species (ROS), activation of oncogenes and cell-cell fusion. The number of senescent cells in tissues rises substantially during normal aging. Although senescent cells can no longer replicate, they remain metabolically active and commonly adopt an immunogenic phenotype consisting of a pro-inflammatory secretome.

8. stem cell exhaustion, wherein a decrease in the renewal of stem cells leads to age-related disorders. This marker is a consequence of DNA damage, deregulated nutrient sensing,

senescence, and other processes already mentioned—in other words, it might be argued that it is not an isolative *true* marker.

9. altered intercellular communication, wherein ageing, compromised cells show an increase in 'self-preserving signals' that result in damage elsewhere. Altered intercellular communication with ageing contributes to decline in tissue health. Like the decline in stem cell renewal, the age-dependent changes in intercellular communication are integrated effects of the other hallmarks of ageing. In particular, senescent cells trigger chronic inflammation that can further damage tissues

10. Oxidation damage to cellular contents caused by 'free radicals', as Oxidative stress this reflects an imbalance between the systemic manifestation of reactive oxygen species and a the body's ability to readily detoxify the reactive intermediates or to repair the resulting damage. Disturbances in the normal redox state of cells can cause toxic effects through the production of peroxides and free radicals that damage all components of the cell, including proteins, lipids, and DNA. Oxidative stress from oxidative metabolism causes base damage, as well as DNA. This is mostly indirect, and caused by reactive oxygen species (ROS) generated, e.g. O_2^- (superoxide radical), OH (hydroxyl radical) and H_2O_2 (hydrogen peroxide). Some reactive oxidative species also act as cellular messengers in redox signaling and can cause disruptions in normal mechanisms of cellular signaling.. Oxidative stress is thought to be involved in the development of many disease processes of consequence to the ageing process including, cancers, Alzheimer's

disease, atherosclerosis, heart failure, and myocardial infarction.

Some of these ten markers or 'mechanisms' can be manipulated [managed] now to inhibit the stress on the body due to ageing. Here we will address what has been shown to be effective.

Directions to Intercept and Challenge Ageing

There are seven processes under active scientific enquiry to retard or reverse ageing. These works include:

1. Nuclear mutations/epimutations are changes to the nuclear DNA (nDNA), or to proteins which bind to the nDNA. Certain mutations can lead to cancer. This would need to be corrected in order to prevent or cure cancer. SENS focuses on a strategy called "whole-body interdiction of lengthening telomeres" (WILT), which would be made possible by periodic regenerative medicine treatments.

2. Mitochondrial mutations influence ageing. Mitochondria are components in our cells that are important for energy production. Because of the highly oxidative environment in mitochondria and their lack of the sophisticated repair systems, mitochondrial mutations are believed to be a major cause of progressive cellular degeneration. This would be corrected by allotopic expression— copying the DNA for mitochondria completely within the cellular nucleus, where it is better protected. De Grey argues that experimental evidence demonstrates that the operation is feasible, however, a 2003 study showed that some

mitochondrial proteins are too hydrophobic to survive the transport from the cytoplasm to the mitochondria

3. Our cells are constantly breaking down proteins and other molecules that are no longer useful or which can be harmful. Those molecules which can't be digested accumulate as junk inside our cells, which is detected in the form of lipofuscin granules. Atherosclerosis, macular degeneration, liver spots on the skin and all kinds of neurodegenerative diseases (such as Alzheimer's disease) are associated with this problem. Junk inside cells might be removed by adding new enzymes to the cell's natural digestion organ, the lysosome. These enzymes would be taken from bacteria, molds and other organisms that are known to completely digest animal bodies.

4. Harmful junk protein can accumulate outside of our cells. Junk here means useless things accumulated by a body, but which cannot be digested or removed by its processes, such as the amyloid plaques characteristic of Alzheimer's disease and other amyloidoses. Junk outside cells might be removed by enhanced phagocytosis (the normal process used by the immune system), and small drugs able to break chemical beta-bonds. The large junk in this class can be removed surgically.

5. Some of the cells in our bodies cannot be replaced or can be only replaced very slowly—more slowly than they die. This decrease in cell number affects some of the most important tissues of the body. Muscle cells are lost in skeletal muscles and the heart, causing them to become frailer with age. Loss of neurons in the substantia nigra causes

Parkinson's disease, while loss of immune cells impairs the immune system. This can currently be partly corrected by therapies involving exercise and growth factors, but stem cell therapy, regenerative medicine and tissue engineering are almost certainly required for any more than just partial replacement of lost cells.

6. Senescence is a phenomenon where the cells are no longer able to divide, but also do not die and let others divide. They may also do other harmful things, like secreting proteins. Degeneration of joints, immune senescence, accumulation of visceral fat and type 2 diabetes are caused by this. Cells sometimes enter a state of resistance to signals sent, as part of a process called apoptosis, to instruct cells to destroy themselves. Cells in this state could be eliminated by forcing them to apoptose (via suicide genes, vaccines, or recently discovered senolytic agents), and healthy cells would multiply to replace them.

7. Cells are held together by special linking proteins. When too many cross-links form between cells in a tissue, the tissue can lose its elasticity and cause problems including arteriosclerosis, presbyopia and weakened skin texture. These are chemical bonds between structures that are part of the body, but not within a cell. In senescent people many of these become brittle and weak.

Leaping Toward Life Extension

It may be simplistic, but in later life we suffer from life-shortening circumstances - from vulnerability to accidents and age-related chronic disease such as cancer or cardiovascular disease; all of which introduce mortality. Extension of expected lifespan can be advanced by eight simple adult 'choices':

1. Avoid accident producing environments [e.g. risk sports]
2. Daily monitoring of health markers [e.g. pulse, blood pressure, weight change]
3. Access improved and *regular* medical care,
4. Obtain vaccinations,
5. Foster and maintain good nutrition consistent with the body's needs, environment and exertion,
6. Limit caloric intake, reduce body-fat
7. Engage in regular repetitive exercise
8. Avoid self-generated hazards [e.g. smoking]

A more comprehensive step by step programme will follow in Chapters __ through ___. Before getting stymied by ethics, brain reward systems, goals and habituation action is suggested. Start with a combination of the eight above. Start walking or jogging [more?], curb your known impulse dietary indiscretions, quit smoking, stay away from bungee jumps, monitor your weight and blood pressure-pulse and see a Physician at the very least. We'll go further – further along.

Money and Simple Choices

Conspicuously missing from the list of choices is perhaps the most dramatically important consideration – money. Wealth and specifically 'disposable income' appears more and more essential to accommodate life extension efforts. In North America access to advanced [radical and contemporary] medical care has become unattainable for most people because of cost. This is also true of access to nutritional supplementation and psychiatric or psychological support. Just 'staying healthy' has become out of reach for many, even among the upper decile of the middle class.

There are two apparent methods of rectifying this; political will to lower the costs of goods and service by regulation [e.g. socializing advanced medicine which is more often than not considered 'elective' and the financial burden of the patient - and socialized pharmacological nutrition supplementation]. The only alternative to bending political will is to secure the money to pay the 'going price', through whatever means are possible. For those at the end of their working life and facing 'retirement', the latter seems unreasonable. What price do we, as a culture, place on continuing health and well-being of those who are late in their lives.

Non-human Successes

Widely recognized successful methods of extending maximum lifespan has been realized in 'modelling' organisms such as nematodes, fruit flies, and small mammals [e.g. laboratory mice]. Successes have been seen in studies which employ:

- caloric restriction,
- gene manipulation, and
- administration of pharmaceuticals.

Extrapolation of these to humans has found many adherents, though thorough testing of each has been limited in scope. Using evolutionary pressures such as breeding from only older members of a species or altering levels of extrinsic mortality have been studied. It is noteworthy that some animals such as hydra, flatworms, and certain sponges, corals, and jellyfish do not die of old age and exhibit potential immortality; and the underlying reasons for those circumstances are actively being investigated to determine if a transference to human biology is attainable.

The Ethics of Life-Extension

Late twentieth and early twenty-first century scholarship has danced around the ethics of 'radical' forms of human life extension, in some instances arguing that such interventions will make the species less evolvable, which would be morally undesirable. What constitutes a 'radical technology of life-extension, and what is 'mainstream' technology for life perpetuation. There may be empirical and evaluative claims in support of the argument about radical methods, but we must be reminded that at one time vaccination was a radical idea – and its universalisation made it low tech and available aa a mainstream technology – all intended to prolong the life and health of the individual vaccinated.

Radical increases in life expectancy could, in principle, reduce the evolutionary potential of human populations through both biological and cultural mechanisms. It has been asserted that if life extension did reduce the evolvability of the species, this will be undesirable for three reasons:

- it may increase the species' susceptibility to extinction risks,
- it may adversely affect institutions and practices that promote well-being, and

- it may impede moral progress.

The wish to extend the human lifespan has a long tradition in many cultures. Optimistic views of the possibility of achieving this goal through the latest developments in medicine feature increasingly in serious scientific and philosophical discussion. Focusing on interventions in biological ageing, one can distinguish between research that is first and foremost aimed at prolonging life by slowing or even arresting ageing processes and research that is directed at combating the diseases that seem to be intrinsically connected with biological ageing. Generally Medical ethicist are not opposed to the latter interventions but grind away against the first which focuses on increasing human life expectancy beyond the average as a primary goal, merely because there exists, as Glannon puts it, "the deeper conviction that there is intrinsic value in living much longer than we presently do, given that being alive is intrinsically valuable". There are at least two agendae at work in this 'ethic', that life-prolongation is not in the interest of those who cater to illness and a culture of 'health care provision', and there must be some fundamental difference between the desirability of being alive (within the limits of the 'average life expectancy') and the desirability of being alive beyond those limits. In the case desirability of life, we deal with the possession and continuation of something we have a right to maintain.

Ethics Compared to Limits on Freedoms and Interventions

Ethical 'difficulties' encountered in navigating between different perspectives on human life-enhancement are structurally similar to those that figure in perennial debates in political philosophy, specifically as it applies to how states should balance individual liberties against the common good, and about the limits of paternalistic intervention to prevent individuals from making choices severely detrimental to their own welfare. This is, some suggest, precisely how ethical questions about enhancement should be approached. Benefits and possible hidden costs of new technologies ought not to be weighted as if they were nothing more than a novel gamble that individuals may consider playing for themselves. Such gambles may play out well or badly for the individual. The situation of choice that everyone will find themselves inexorably drawn into -- when another extending technology is realised – becomes whether that situation is something to promote, or instead to try to resist. Within this ethic there is a third option; neutrality – neither opposing or endorsing research and development geared to life-extending technologies.

One class of potential human enhancement technology that calls for ethical scrutiny is life-extension technology. If it becomes possible to extend people's lives *far* beyond their current duration, this will be a profound change in the conditions of human existence, and there is an historical record in support [the first wave technologies]. While there are certainly great distributional injustices that could arise in the face of such technology, it is considerably more dilute to propose that life-extension would represent a poison-pill for those who have access to the relevant technology. The benefits of an increased healthy lifespan to individual users are plain to see. Attempts to identify harms to users caused by their increasing lifespans typically devolve into hazy and unpersuasive talk about the importance of 'the given', or about the moral hazards of hubris. In *Humanity's End: Why We Should Reject Radical Enhancement* (2010), Ethicist Nicholas Agar argues that radically extending our lives – will result in people's lives being "completely dominated by the fear of death". Agar's argument starts from the individual user's perspective. He maintains that it would be a 'bad thing' for the individual to opt for negligible senescence [The term first used in the early 1990s by Caleb Finch described organisms such as lobsters and hydras, which do not show symptoms of ageing. "Engineered negligible senescence" first appeared in 1999 and sparked an approach to the science of ageing, and "an effort to expand regenerative medicine into the territory of ageing". The term now encompasses seven categories of ageing "damage" and a specific regenerative medical proposal for treating each].

If it really would be bad for individuals (by their own volition) to undertake radical life-extension treatment, why not trust people to not do what is injurious for them by their own measurement? One argument is motivated by anticipation of the emergence of a destructive economy of desire and incentive where radical life-extension has become an option, and where individuals have been left to decide for themselves – as some, like Agar, prefer in principle – whether they will pursue it. Indeed, the corrosive fear of death that is central to Agar's argument may enter the frame not only once a person has actively undertaken to extend her life, but as soon as the option to significantly extend her life becomes available. If the fear of death will spoil people's lives in an era of negligible senescence, there are normative implications in this not only for individuals – of the 'buyer beware' type that Agar emphasises –but for legislatures, voters, funding bodies, and researchers, insofar as all of these can shape the potentially perilous situation we eventually find ourselves in regarding the prospect of radical life-extension. Given that life-extension technologies are already being researched in earnest; it may come as a relief to find that Agar's argument from fear of death, while it is a significant improvement on previous ethical arguments against radical life-extension, ultimately remains unconvincing.

Religious Convictions and Life-Extension

The most commonly cited argument is that life extension as an explicit aim is contrary to the wisdom of ages as contained in various religious and non-religious spiritual traditions. Although all traditions agree that life is worthy and should not be taken (without good reason, or at all), there is always a notion that human beings miss the essence of life by focusing on the preservation of their self or "ego". The argument pursues the premise that wrong self-preservation is reflected in life-preservation as advanced by the advocates of life-extension. The connectivity is tenuous.

Many spiritual and religious traditions make a point that truly human life by the decentring of the self. In the Christian tradition, as expressed by Thomas Aquinas, for example, the notion of eternal life does not refer primarily to a prolongation of earthly life based on the conception of an immortal soul; rather, it refers to the fullness of a human life that can be reached to the extent that one's goal in life is no longer the preservation of the self, but the communion with and service to God and one's neighbour. The argument, stripped of varnish is that service to God and others is the focus of life to the exclusion of self. This is untenable because service or 'works as defined scripturally cannot be done when one is dead. The preservation of the person, physical and psychically is required in order for service (which is meritorious in all Western religions) to be carried out. Life extension merely extends the opportunity for service. The same sentiment for extended service to God and man is in fact been advanced in other monotheistic religions, such as Judaism and Islam. Within Eastern spirituality, we see that Hinduism, Buddhism and explicitly non-religious spiritual approaches all point to the importance of letting go of the ego. While less concentrated upon service to man these disciplines do concentrate on the development of spiritual insight – and set rigorous guidelines for pursuing this over the maximum time available to the individual adherent.

It has been proposed that these traditions maintain that the more one's self is de-Centred, the more one loses interest in self-preservation or extension of the biological lifespan. There is however no innate command that seeking the flourishing of other people (a sign both of happiness and a meaningful life) precludes 'self-flourishing' which will yield further opportunity for the former.

That the world's spiritual traditions are worth listening to, because they are a rich and often ancient source of experience with the living of a meaningful life in various cultural contexts. When the wisdom of these different contexts converges, it seems likely that something of importance may appear. They each make us aware that quality of life is not simply in the length of lifetime; but in what proportion, for whatever is the psychical and physical length of life afforded – that man takes of every opportunity for service and devotion to God and/or others.

It has been challenged that the wisdom of the spiritual traditions is inspired by the fact that human beings have to cope with their mortality and seek an escape in transcendence. Although it may be true that this motivation is present among the followers of diverse spiritual traditions, some muse that the traditions themselves are too sophisticated and well thought through to be accused of escapism. It is argued elsewhere that there is a secular parallel to the experience of the de-centering of the self as related to the experience of life's meaning.

The Inequity Ethical Argument

One obvious moral problem is the already existing "unequal death" when perceived across a global 'playing field'. As Mauron argues, this inequality, which is observed in the counterpoint of both the First World to the Third World - and between rich and poor within Western welfare societies, is the main ethical obstacle. How can we justify trying to extend the lives of those who have more already?

The figures speak for themselves: in a number of African countries south of the Sahara, life expectancy is less than 40 years. The average lifespan in rich and developed countries is now exceeds 80 years. The causes of this inequality exceed the strictly medical realm. It is mainly the combination of illness with poverty that is responsible for this mortality in under-developed areas. Global inequality ought not to not present a problem for bioethics. Disparities are acknowledged as scandalously unfair but are the precinct pf responsible and responsive governments and non-governmental organisations, not of bioethicists. Bioethicists may focus on morally relevant complex interrelation between the health of populations and international justice. Efforts to counter the march of bioethics toward a subsystem of applied ethics which became dominant starting in the 1970s. In a globalizing world, problems of ill health in the undeveloped nations are related to how the developed and wealthy nations use their political, financial and scientific powers. Contemporary bioethics, therefore, cannot limit itself to how and under what conditions new scientific developments may be applied but must also confront the question whether these developments contribute to a more just world. Exactly the same demands must be placed on how well all nations use new scientific developments towards life-extension in a more just and expanding world.

The principle of distributive justice argument against life extension was formulated along utilitarian lines by Harris, among others. The fact that western medicine has no means to treat all patients is no argument to qualify it as 'unjust' to treat some of them. Harris maintains: "If immortality or increased life expectancy is a good, it is doubtful ethics to deny palpable goods to some people because we cannot provide them for all". Davis defends the same conclusion, using slightly different reasoning. To deny the Haves a treatment that they can afford because the Have-nots cannot afford it "is justified only if doing so makes the Have-nots more than marginally better off". The burden for the Have-nots of the availability of life-extending treatments for the Haves has much less 'alleged weigh if then compared with the number of additional life years that the Haves would lose if life extension were prevented from becoming available.

Both utilitarian arguments are problematic in two respects. In the first place, they make no distinction between the right of Haves to maintain what they already have, such as certain medical treatments for age-related diseases, and the right to become Have-mores through research and development to enhance the total lifespan. This fundamental difference between the real and the potential may entertain moral repercussions in the light of applied 'justice'. Treatments that exist in reality but are not available to all raise questions of distributive justice. Potential treatments, it is asserted, require prior questions: for what goals are they developed? are they worthwhile at all, and for whom? who will profit? who will be harmed? In the second place, by calculating only benefits and burdens, or burdens of different weights, they neglect the moral quality of certain states of affairs that can be considered wrong and unjust *in se and* should be prevented from becoming even more wrong or unjust. The position is then that life extension research and development bypasses the noteworthy 'moral principles' of equity and integrity. By focusing on how to justify the distribution of means that are not available to all, we sideline the whole issue of inequality in opportunities. The original problem of why some can be treated and others cannot be not considered. With regard to extending lifespan, the medical establishment maintains we are not dealing with treatments but with the question of the desirability of research and development, and, consequently, of financial investments that will not diminish these global inequalities in life expectancy, or, even worse, may increase them.

Prolonging life, therefore they emphasise, ought not to be segregates from the more fundamental question of integrity: given the problem of unequal death, can the global culture morally afford to invest in research to extend life? The contemporary agenda of bioethics happens to be largely defined by dilemmas and problems raised by Western medicine and biomedical research. Some medical ethicist has framed a question that it may be relevant to know the opinions on life-extension technology of all those people whose risk of dying before the age of 40 could be diminished by 'lesser and fairer' simple, low-technology means.

Social Otherness Arguments

Life is always life with others, even when it is extended. How this relatedness to others is interpreted may be the focus for ethical considerations wherein human beings are perceived as primarily individuals, related to each other by contract and negotiations, and motivated by self-interest. The other person has an instrumental value, and can appear as a friend, a competitor or even an enemy. The sum of all others, incorporated in the community or society, fulfils a merely instrumental value: the community or society is judged by the extent to which it facilitates its members to realise their individual life plan. In such a view, the good life is the good life *for the me*, defined and measured by myself. Autonomy and authenticity are central values. Arguments in favour of life extension are often based on the presuppositions of such perceptions of interface.

In contrast, communitarian anthropology views human beings social beings: relations with others belong to the essentials of what it is to live a human life. The social context in this schema is not just an instrumental means to realize individual life plans, but the precondition for living a human life. Human beings are seen not to thrive and be alive without meaningful relations with others. Goods that are essential for a good life, such as friendship, are essentially goods that are bound to the social dimensions of life.

With respect to biological ageing, the two anthropological views have been manipulated to be symbiotic or combined. In the still-hypothetical situation that extending biological age becomes a medical–technical option, it is primarily a matter of autonomy whether a subject wants to choose it. This freedom of choice fits with the first perspective [life as me]. The communitarian view, however, stresses the importance of the social network as a condition without parallel for a truly human life. This is seen, not a simple psychical condition [in the sense that I feel better with others] but an ethical one: in order to realize a morally good life, I have to realize myself as a community being. Being with others as such is considered intrinsically valuable, not the fact that the other is "useful" for my purposes. This would appear to exclude the option that an extension of biological age is intrinsically valuable. It is valuable only if it also extends our life as communal beings. Living longer is valuable only if it results in living longer in meaningful relations. Quality of time outweighs quantity of time. The real ethical challenge for ageing societies, therefore, should be how to improve the conditions for life as a life in community, and not how to stop ageing as such. The tenuous nature of the argument is a presupposition that the extended life is available to the few not the many as a hypothetical condition [predicated on research not even yet contemplated], and further assumes that those with extended lives will refuse to serve the collective good in proportion to the extent demanded of those 'alive; at any age.

Ethical Theorists

The three principal arguments offered differ in cogency. The argument of spiritual tradition is most spoken of; though it is not convincing, particularly to those who do not 'adhere' to the tradition. The argument pandering to injustice is the strongest, because it has a common-sense argumentative force that is recognised in most ethical theories. The argument citing the social nature of human beings, derives its cogency from the willingness to critically consider and complete the presuppositions of one's moral theory.

If the three arguments are read seamlessly it is emphasised that they are complementary and endorse one another, in the sense that those who search for a meaningful life in the diminution of the self will thereby acknowledge the importance of the community and champion a lop-sided form of global justice.

Much of the literature on the ethics of life-extension simply deals in discussion and conjecture about the future

prospects of the relevant technologies. At the modest end of the spectrum there are authors who
consider the possibility of typical lifespans and healthspans increasing to approximately double their current length (Singer 1991; Glannon 2002a; Walker 2007). At the more speculative end of the spectrum, others advert to the possibility of lives extended towards 1000 years, or even extended indefinitely, i.e. not to the point of immortality as such, but as long as possible within the constraints imposed by (i) finite material resources, (ii) fatal accidents and (iii) the finite lifespan of the universe.5 An assortment of technological advances have been identified as potential routes towards dramatically extended human life. At the genetic level, the hope is that it will become possible to manipulate the telomere nucleotide
sequences at the ends of chromosomes, which regulate chromosome replication, and whose normal deterioration over time induces cellular senescence. The reversal of ageing effects in mice has already been achieved via this route (Jaskelioff et al. 2011), and together with other novel advances – e.g. in hormone therapy, or caloric restriction, or synthetically produced bodily organs – this development raises the
possibility of a dramatically extended human lifespan (see Marshall 2006; Barazetti 2011). We do not pretend to have the expertise required to assess the likelihood of the predictions we find in the literature.

Wrapping up arguments in a flag of moral authority argues that no individual should have the option for life extension if science progresses enough to offer it. The focus here is on the ethics of 'investing' in research aimed at further life extension. Since such research has an institutional aspect related to public funding, this aspect requires thorough reflection and dialogue by biogerontologists and their scientific-organizations, by ethicists and philosophers, and by society at large - those who are directly affected thereby. A reasonable question must be framed that contains the contingency of 'to what extent life extension contributes to the public good'. This is ambiguous. It comes close to "public interest", which some frame as the aggregate of individual private interests of individuals. As opposed to this, the concept of the common good entails a society where individuals inextricably bind up their own good with the good of the whole. It forces reflection on the question of whether living longer is good for me as a human being, and whether a society whose members have a much longer life than is the case at present would be a better society.

A reply to both communalist and other objections to life extension is that issues of meaning and of communities are highly personal matters: in both domains, people have to find their own position and it is posited focally, possess the right to free choice. Personal answers and choices can be enriched by being embedded in traditions of wisdom with regard to how to live a human live. It is this embedding that many intend to add to the discussion on life-extending research. With regard to a better society, in a globalizing world as ours is, there is a moral challenge to expand our view of the common good to encompass good for all, worldwide by extending the lives of all.

Extension inevitably raises the question of whether we can morally afford *now*, as a question of moral integrity, to invest time and money in researching and implementing technologies to extend all men's lives - while refuting the short-term issue of unequal death which, as we have seen, is an untenable premise. The issue becomes one of public will, or if you can view it as such - of political will; to invest in the future of man.

We have seen that ethics of stumbling toward life extension are complicated by issues such as inequity. However, we must accept that life-prolongation is being creatively done by millions of people who are 'looking after themselves with a long-range view of their lives'. Research on ageing retardation or reversal is going forward at a rapid pace and many of its technologies are dropping from 'radical', 'elective' and expensive into the mainstream of medical practice.

The Brain, the Reward System and Well-Being

The nature of the brain's influence on goals and habituation geared to life-prolongation will appear more complex in vocabulary but less daunting in 'skepticism' than the ethics issues were.

Shaping Goals

Goals are what keeps us going. Often, we hear of someone retiring after 40 years of work-orientation - and dropping dead within a few short weeks. Once we lose our momentum, and our direction, we are in trouble. The drive or motivator considered here is life-extension. It has been observed that a person is generally happiest when in the middle of the project, and not at the end of it. Frequently the situation arises at the conclusion of a consuming project when the individual immediately looks around for something else to do. The next project is expected to yield contentment primarily in its execution (which results in a rewarding elation).

It is human nature to develop goals. We can't live without them, or at least, not for very long; therefore, if you don't have yourself a list right at this moment - it's important step to start keyboarding. If possible start with an Excel spreadsheet which can be expanded or collapsed from a list to a detailed plan for happiness. The section below on Goal Analysis and Practice gives some elements of a start-up list, which can be augmented with personally selected goals. People who are successful see a wrong direction as a valuable learning experience while unsuccessful, categorically unhappy people see a wrong direction as a failure.

Precession

Buckminster Fuller, (1895-1983) an American philosopher, architect, humanitarian, visionary, inventor and author developed one of the century's most creative approaches when he wrote of the "law of precession" as part of the goal setting process The Law of Precession is the Universal Law that says "nothing moves until something "acts"." In other words, it's the law of action. No goal is 'real' unless acted upon, but the work must overcome inertia, with one foot in front of the other.

The law of precession also maintains that any action, such as a rock thrown into a still pond, not only creates ripples of waves in the water, the waves also spread out and continue to contact and meet other waves, rocks and may even reach the distant shore, making changes along the way. For the purposes here, we will define the ripples as 'side effects' since they operate on a different axis from the goal. In other words, action not only creates momentum, the correct action which is also intended for the "greater good" of mankind, also has a *synergistic* effect on the rest of the universe. The amplification of good by successive actions may result in exponential social improvement and social contentedness. This is a preferential universal circumstance, and an admirable influence resulting from any improved individual's happiness.

The law of precession is arguably the most underutilized of all the Universal Laws, because everyone that initially becomes aware of the law of attraction, thinks that its manifestation is all magical, *"hocus-pocus"* and that it's not supposed to take any *real effort.*

Compared, say, to the laws of attraction or mathematics - the law of precession ends up being the, "poor relation*"* of the universal laws, because this is where the *"work"* comes in; a word most of us don't want to hear, *or do*!

In today's technologically-manipulated, computer-managed society, everyone wants to wait it out for a rosy outcome. But, without the "action" part of the equation, there are not likely to be results. The law of precession explains the effect that "bodies in motion" have on other, "bodies in motion."

Don't *wait* for the law of attraction to bring results. Take positive action on your thoughts, dreams and ideas, but most importantly on your *intuitions.* That is the best indicator of *when* and what *type* of action to take. It is a principle which always ensures that we gain many things beyond the actual goal in itself. Most importantly; it is not reaching the goal - but what we learn and how much we grow along the way towards it. The over-riding motivator to extend healthy life requires stepping forward.

Acute and Chronic Experience

Positive and negative experiences fall into two broad categories: those that are acute events (e.g., death of a loved one) and chronic, daily experiences (e.g. health challenges); and both influence satisfaction reports. Tal Ben-Shahar, an author and lecturer at Harvard University, asserts that happiness should be people's ultimate goal, the primary factor in evaluating alternative choices. This 'work' of choice and action presumes that life is to continue, and the presumption foreshadows all goal setting. As an ultimate goal this implies, getting 'happier' with pursuit of immediate joyful experience in ways that contribute to more long-term, meaningful satisfaction. Furthermore, Ben-Shahar argues that pursuing genuine self-motivated goals, rather than just instant pleasure or selflessness in service of long delayed enjoyment, results in an optimal combination of short- and long-term happiness. Contentment can be closely associated with the concept of happiness and satisfaction.

Wide spectrum satisfaction can reflect experiences that have influenced a person in a positive way. These experiences have the ability to self-motivate people to pursue and reach their goals. There are two kinds of emotions that may influence how people perceive their lives. Hope and optimism both consist of cognitive processes that are usually oriented towards achievement of goals and the perception of those goals. This indicated that positive views and life satisfaction were completely mediated by the concept of self-esteem, together with the different ways in which ideas and events are perceived by people. It is crucial that this floor of satisfaction be in place for life extension goals and habituation to be successful. Several studies found that self-esteem plays a definite role in influencing life satisfaction. There is also a homeostatic model that supports these findings. A person's mood and outlook on past and future life can also influence their perception of their own life satisfaction.

It is proffered that wide spectrum satisfaction comes from within an individual; based on the individual's personal values and what he or she holds important. For some it is healthy personal actualisation, for others it is love, and for others it is money or other material items; either way, it varies from one person to another.

Materialism as a Ground

Economic materialism can be considered a value. Several researchers attest that materialistic individuals were predominantly male, and that materialistic people reported a lower life satisfaction level than their non-materialistic peers. The same is true of people who value their finances over helping other people. This is because the money they have can buy them the assets they deem valuable. Materialistic people are less satisfied with life because they constantly want more and more belongings, and once those belongings are obtained they lose value, which in turn causes these people to want more belongings, perpetuating the cycle. If these materialistic individuals do not have enough money to satisfy their craving for more items, they become more dissatisfied. This has been referred to as a hedonic treadmill. If an individual does not hold the acquisition of wealth as a high priority, his or her personal financial state will not make a difference on how happy he or she is with life. Individuals reporting a high value on traditions [and religion] reported a higher level of life satisfaction. Perceiving life prolongation as a function of these traditions has already been discussed, and such people readily see 'self-flourishing' as an improved opportunity to serve their fellows [and their God as they envision it]. In contrast materialists are marshalling everything to tend and expand things to the exclusion of life actualization.

Other individuals that reported higher levels of overall satisfaction were people who valued creativity, and people who valued respect for and from others—two more qualities seemingly not related to material goods. Acculturation of deeply held beliefs affects the subjective well-being and motivation toward self-preservation. Well-being includes both general life satisfaction, and the relative balance of positive affect versus negative affect in daily life. Culture directs the attention to different sources of information for making the life satisfaction judgements, thus affecting subjective well-being appraisal. Any deeply held belief can be challenged, rewritten and habituated with proper technique – but it is a daunting task.

Individualistic cultures {which focus on self-generated action) direct attention to inner states and feelings (such as positive or negative affects), while in collectivistic cultures the attention is directed to outer sources (i.e. adhering to social norms or fulfilling one's duties). Suh et al. (1998) found that the correlation between life satisfaction and the prevalence of positive affect is higher in individualistic cultures, whereas in collectivistic cultures affect and adhering to norms are equally important for life satisfaction.

'Subjective well-being' may be defined in three parts:
- How much positive emotion (positive affect) as opposed to negative emotion (negative affect) does a person have, and
- how one views one's life overall (wide spectrum satisfaction)
- What level of 'hope' for the future exists

Positive psychology finds it very important to study contributes to people 'flourishing' and finds it just as important to focus on the constructive ways in which people function and adapt to present and future, as opposed to the general field of psychology which focuses more on what goes wrong or is pathological with human beings. The field of computational psychiatry is currently leading this study. That discipline is also closely identified with studies in artificial intelligence.

Intuiting Decisions on Longevity Goals

In our daily lives, we usually weigh multiple criteria implicitly and we may be comfortable with the consequences of such decisions that are made based on only intuition. Without recourse to assessment, intuition is the ability to acquire knowledge without proof, evidence, or conscious reasoning, or without understanding how the knowledge was acquired. Different writers give the word "intuition" a great variety of different meanings, ranging from direct access to unconscious knowledge, unconscious cognition, inner sensing, inner insight to unconscious pattern-recognition and the ability to understand something instinctively, without the need for conscious reasoning.

Desire: The Lead-in to Brain Bio-Chemistry

Gratification is the pleasurable reaction in measured direct response to a *fulfillment* of a desire or goal. Desire is a sense of longing or hoping for a person, object, or outcome. Here we are considering desire as effected by two of the three, the object which is extended lifespan, and the outcome which is the resultant [if successful outcome is achieved through goal and habit modification]. The same sense is expressed by emotions such as "craving". When a person desires something or someone, their sense of longing is excited by the enjoyment or the thought of the motivator [e.g. life prolongation], and they want to take actions to obtain their goal. As we will detail later the modification of brain influence through habit modification is a significant way of managing the outcomes of the sought-after desire. The motivational aspect of desire has long been noted by philosophers. Thomas Hobbes (1588–1679) asserted that human desire is the fundamental motivation of *all* human action.

Desires can best be described points of reference, and generally are not directly as focused as are goals - which develop a line of action and time line to their execution. Desires are often classified as emotions by laypersons, but health practitioners usually describe desires as different from emotions; arguing that desires arise from bodily structures [i.e. the stomach's need for food], whereas emotions arise from a person's mental state. The interface between desire as a function of brain bio-chemistry as represented by the rewards system and the mentally developed wanting of an outcome is a subject of much current scholarship.

Desire is at the core of much of literature which often create drama by showing cases where human desire is impeded by social conventions, class, or cultural barrier (and generally these are overcome. David Hume (1711–1776) claimed that desires and passions are non-cognitive, automatic bodily responses, and he argued that reasoning is "capable only of devising means to ends set by [bodily] desire". Immanuel Kant (1724–1804) called any action based on desires a hypothetical imperative, meaning by this that it is a command of reason that applies only if one desires the objective in question.

Brain Contribution to Keying 'Longevity as Desire'

A 2008 study entitled *"The Neural Correlates of Desire"* showed that the human brain categorizes stimuli according to its desirability by activating three different brain areas: the superior orbitofrontal cortex, the mid-cingulate cortex, and the anterior cingulate cortex. Research also shows that the orbitofrontal cortex has connections to both the opioid and dopamine systems, and stimulating this cortex is associated with subjective reports of pleasure. Dopamine confers motivational salience ("wanting") on a reward itself or associated cues (nucleus accumbens shell region), updates the value placed on different goals in light of this new experience (orbital prefrontal cortex), helps consolidate multiple forms of memory (amygdala and hippocampus), and encodes new motor programmes that will facilitate obtaining this reward in the future (nucleus accumbens core region and dorsal striatum). In this example, dopamine modulates the processing of sensorimotor information in diverse neural circuits to maximize the ability of the organism to obtain future rewards"

Gratification, as with all emotions, is a motivator of behaviour - and thus plays a role in the entire range of human social systems. Something concluded positively is gratifying.

Euphoria and Reward

Euphoria is an affective state in which a person experiences pleasure or excitement and intense feelings of well-being and happiness. Certain drugs, many of which are addictive, can cause euphoria, which at least partially motivates their recreational use. Similarly, certain natural rewards and social activities, such as aerobic exercise, laughter, listening to emotionally arousing music, music-making, and dancing, can induce a state of euphoria. Euphoria is also a symptom of certain neurological or neuropsychiatric disorders, such as mania. Elements of the human sexual response cycle are also associated with the induction of euphoria.

Kent Berridge asserts that intense euphoria occurs from the simultaneous activation of every hedonic hotspot within the brain's reward system.

The Rewards System and Salience

The reward system is a group of neural structures responsible for three principal developments:

1. incentive salience (i.e., motivation and "wanting", desire, or craving for a reward),
2. associative learning (primarily positive reinforcement and classical conditioning),
3. positive emotions, particularly ones which involve pleasure as a core component (e.g., joy, euphoria and ecstasy).

Reward is the attractive and motivational property of a stimulus that induces appetitive behaviour, also known as approach behaviour, and consummatory behaviour. In its description of a rewarding stimulus (i.e., "a reward").

Intrinsic rewards are unconditioned rewards that are attractive and motivate behaviour because they are inherently pleasurable. Extrinsic rewards (e.g., money) are conditioned rewards that are attractive and motivate behaviour; but are not inherently pleasurable. Extrinsic rewards derive their motivational value as a result of a learned association (i.e., conditioning) with intrinsic rewards. Extrinsic rewards may also elicit pleasure (e.g., winning a lottery) after being classically conditioned with intrinsic rewards.

Brain 'Workings'

Incentive salience is the "wanting" or "desire" attribute, which includes a motivational component, that is assigned to a rewarding stimulus by the brains nucleus accumbens shell (NAcc shell). The degree of dopamine neurotransmission into that shell from the mesolimbic pathway is highly correlated with the magnitude of incentive salience for rewarding stimuli.

Activation of the dorsorostral region of the nucleus accumbens correlates with increases in wanting, without concurrent increases in liking. Dopaminergic neurotransmission into the nucleus accumbens shell is not only responsible for appetitive motivational salience (i.e., incentive salience) towards rewarding stimuli, but also for aversive motivational salience, which directs behaviour away from undesirable stimuli. D1-type medium spiny neurons within the NAcc shell confer incentive salience for rewarding stimuli, while D2-type medium spiny neurons within the NAcc shell confer aversive motivational salience for undesirable stimuli.

Robinson and Berridge's incentive-sensitization theory (1993) proposed that *reward* contains separable psychological components: wanting (incentive) and liking (pleasure). To explain increasing contact with a certain stimulus such as chocolate, there are two independent factors at work – our desire to have the chocolate (wanting) and the pleasure effect of the chocolate (liking). Wanting and liking are two aspects of the same process, so rewards are usually wanted and liked to the same degree. However, wanting and liking also change independently under certain circumstances.

The brain structures that compose the reward system are located primarily within the cortico-basal ganglia-thalamo-cortical loop; the basal ganglia portion of the loop drives activity within the reward system. Most of the pathways that connect structures within the reward system are founded on four neural sub-systems:

1. glutamatergic interneurons,
2. GABAergic medium spiny neurons, and
3. dopaminergic projection neurons, and
4. other types of projection neurons (e.g., orexinergic projection neurons).

The reward system includes the ventral tegmental area, ventral striatum (i.e., the nucleus accumbens and olfactory tubercle), dorsal striatum (i.e., the caudate nucleus and putamen), substantia nigra (i.e., the pars compacta and pars reticulata), prefrontal cortex, anterior cingulate cortex, insular cortex, hippocampus, hypothalamus (particularly, the orexinergic nucleus in the lateral hypothalamus), thalamus (multiple nuclei), subthalamic nucleus, globus pallidus (both external and internal), ventral pallidum, parabrachial nucleus, amygdala, and the remainder of the extended amygdala. The dorsal raphe nucleus and cerebellum appear to modulate some forms of reward-related cognition (i.e., associative learning, motivational salience, and positive emotions) and behaviours as well.

The reward system contains pleasure centres or hedonic hotspots – i.e., brain structures that mediate pleasure or "liking" reactions from intrinsic rewards. Up through 2015 these hedonic hotspots have been identified in sub-compartments within the nucleus accumbens shell, ventral pallidum, and parabrachial nucleus of the pons; the insular cortex and orbitofrontal cortex likely contain hedonic hotspots as well. Opioid and endocannabinoid, but not dopamine, injections in the ventrorostral region of the nucleus accumbens are able to increase liking, while injection in other regions may produce aversion or wanting, as dopamine microinjections do.

Most of the dopamine pathways (i.e., neurons that use the neurotransmitter dopamine to communicate with other neurons) that project out of the ventral tegmental area are part of the reward system; in these pathways, dopamine acts on D1-like receptors or D2-like receptors - to either stimulate (D1-like) or inhibit (D2-like) the production of cAMP. The GABAergic medium spiny neurons of the striatum are components of the reward system as well. The glutamatergic projection nuclei in the subthalamic nucleus, prefrontal cortex, hippocampus, thalamus, and amygdala connect to other parts of the reward system via glutamate pathways. The medial forebrain bundle, which is a set of many neural pathways that mediate brain stimulation reward (i.e., reward derived from direct electrochemical stimulation of the lateral hypothalamus), is also a component of the reward system.

The dopamine pathway is focal to circuits facilitating reward.

Pleasure as Extrinsic and Intrinsic Reward

Pleasure is a component of reward, but not all rewards are pleasurable (e.g., money does not elicit pleasure unless this response is conditioned/habituated). Elicitation of pleasure from goal development on a dopamine levels is possible; and is being studied now. Stimuli that are naturally pleasurable, and therefore attractive, are known as *intrinsic rewards*, whereas stimuli that are attractive and motivate approach behaviour, but are not inherently pleasurable, are termed *extrinsic rewards*. Extrinsic rewards (e.g., money) are rewarding as a result of a learned association with an intrinsic reward. In other words, extrinsic rewards function as motivational magnets that elicit "wanting", but not "liking" reactions once they have been acquired.

The simultaneous activation of every hedonic hotspot within the entire reward system is believed to be necessary for generating the sensation of an 'euphoria'.

The reward system includes independent processes of wanting and liking. The processes are divisible and are likely carried on by distinct bio-chemical systems in the brain The wanting component is said to be controlled by dopaminergic pathways, whereas the liking component is thought to be controlled by opiate-benzodiazepine systems.

Neurons play a crucial role in motivation, reward-related behaviour, attention, and multiple forms of memory. This organization of the dopamine system (an organic chemical of the catecholamine and phenethylamine families that plays several important roles in the brain and body. It is an amine synthesized by removing a carboxyl group from a molecule of its precursor chemical L-DOPA, which is synthesized in the brain), wide projection from a limited number of cell bodies, permits coordinated responses to potent new rewards. Thus, acting in diverse terminal fields, dopamine confers motivational salience ("wanting") on the reward itself or associated cues (nucleus accumbens shell region), updates the value placed on different goals in light of this new experience (orbital prefrontal cortex), helps consolidate multiple forms of memory (amygdala and hippocampus), and encodes new motor programmes that will facilitate obtaining this reward in the future (nucleus accumbens core region and dorsal striatum). In this example, dopamine modulates the processing of sensorimotor information in diverse neural circuits to maximize the ability of the individual to obtain future rewards.

Habits and Habit-Alteration

Life Extension demands that good habits be introduced [or reinforced] and bad habits broken and displaced. These are 'hard-wired inside the brain's rewards system and need detailed techniques to move them around. Habits which need to be altered for life prolongation which are separate from Nutrition, Supplementation and Exercise are discussed in Book 2 of this series. Habitual behaviour often goes unnoticed in persons exhibiting it, because we do not 'need to engage in self-analysis' when undertaking routine tasks. Habits are sometimes compulsory. New behaviours can become automatic through the process of habit formation. Old habits are hard to break and new habits are hard to form because the behavioural patterns which humans repeat become imprinted in neural pathways, but it is possible to form new habits through repetition.

When behaviours are repeated in a consistent context, there is an incremental increase in the link between the context and the action. This increases the automaticity of the behaviour in that context. Features of an automatic behaviour reflect either all or some of:

- efficiency
- lack of awareness
- unintentionality
- uncontrollability

Habit formation is the process by which a behaviour, through regular repetition, becomes automatic or habitual. This process of *habit formation can be slow, frequently within a range of 18–254 days (with an average of 60 days).*

As the habit is forming, it can be analysed in three parts:
1. the cue,
2. the behaviour, and
3. the reward.

The cue is the thing that causes the habit to come about, the trigger of the habitual behaviour. This could be anything that one's mind associates with that habit and one will automatically let a habit come to the surface. The behaviour is the actual habit that one exhibits, and the reward, a positive feeling, therefore continues the "habit loop". A habit may initially be triggered by a goal, but over time that goal becomes less necessary and the habit becomes more automatic.

A variety of digital tools, online or mobile apps, have been introduced that are designed to support habit formation. A recent review of such tools, however, suggests most are poorly designed with respect to theory and fail to support the development of automaticity.

Some habits are known as "keystone habits", and these influence-associate the formation of other habits. For example, identifying as the type of person who takes care of their body and is in the habit of exercising regularly, can also influence habits of eating better or using credit cards less often. In business, safety can be a keystone habit that influences other habits that result in greater productivity.

Unlike consciously intended behaviour, which proceeds via a cognitively effortful reflective processing system, behaviour that is directed by habit is regulated by an impulsive processing system, and so can be elicited with minimal cognitive effort, awareness, control, or intention. The habit formation process involves a gradual transfer of action-initiation from the conscious attentional or motivational processes (involved in reflective processing), to external cuing mechanisms characteristic of impulsive processing. Behaviour thus becomes detached from motivational or volitional control, freeing finite cognitive resources for unfamiliar or otherwise more demanding tasks. Upon encountering associated situations, habitual tendencies dominate action regulation, and alternative actions become less readily accessible.

Habit theory proposes that habit strength will predict the likelihood of enactment of habitual behaviour, and that strong habitual tendencies will dominate over any 'broken record' is essentially self-hypnosis into automatic response of incantation of specific formulae in specific circumstances, but it is a self-hypnosis that gets projected, by repetition, into conditioning the nervous system of anyone who happens to come within range of it. The self-centred world views projected by broken record should not be allowed to pass unchallenged - otherwise, by persistence, they will become predominant. Hence dealing specifically with this problem - a problem which roots in conscious, selfish conditioned behaviour. The repetition of a simple pattern ad nauseum until that pattern becomes entrenched in the neuronic structure of the person using it and, in some circumstances, the people who hear it. Getting 'into the habit' may be crucial to achieving or perpetuating appropriate behaviours. Evidence of these effects, albeit predominantly observational and correlational, has been found for many everyday socially significant and health-relevant behaviours, such as physical activity, healthy eating, alcohol consumption, TV viewing, and travel mode choice. Such findings have stimulated interest in habit formation as a behaviour change mechanism. Some have argued that adding habit formation components into behaviour change interventions should sustain what are otherwise typically only short-term effects, by shielding new behaviours against potential motivational lapses.

Habit-based interventions differ from non-habit-based interventions in that they include elements that promote context-dependent repetition, with the explicit aim of developing situation-action associations, and thus, situationally cued automatic behavioural responses. A wealth of habit-based behaviour change interventions have been studied in clinical trials and have mostly shown positive effects on behaviour.

The influence of initial goal-orientation or motivation to alter behaviour through 'modelled' habit-formation remains under-studied. As an intervention strategy, habit formation has been shown to be acceptable to intervention recipients, who report that, through repetition, behaviours gradually become routinized and "second nature."

Nearly half of what you do each day is repetitive behaviour. No matter how invested you are in your goals, taking consistent action to change your habits is both difficult and long-term contingent. There is 'safety' in going back to old thinking and behaviours. You must take deliberate, consistent actions repeatedly over time to defy your brain - if you want to achieve the longevity modelling results you desire. The impetus to create different outcomes is not enough to sustain change. To create new habits, your brain needs consistent evidence that your goal is achievable and worth the effort. Without consistent evidence, your brain will fabricate rationalizations for not changing, and give you reasons for decreasing the value of the goal. You forget why the goal is so important unless you have a monitor (feedback loop) to help you see your way through these typical blocks to progress.

The brain's primary function is to protect you from harm and discomfort, and then to effect improvement in well-being through its rewards system. You must convince your brain that you will not only be safe if you change, you will be better off. To convince your brain, you must compose easily attainable steps that you will repeat for a period of time until they comfortably fit into your routine. You need visual or auditory cues (reminders) that there is a feel-good payoff for the change you want to make. Then every day, you want to recognize every time your remembered and tried to meet your commitment, even if the attempt was small. You have to show your brain that you will succeed, little by little over time.

Behavioural Plan Execution

The key to transformation choices becoming long-lasting behavioural change is to motivate change through:

1. Use pictures and notes to visually remind yourself of what you want to create.

2. Planning and repeating small shifts in behaviour; so, you can see early and consistent evidence that you are successful.

3. Document the evidence of each positive step when you journal and dialogue about your progress.

First, make sure you define specific activities you can celebrate. Chunk your goal into small action-nodes that will move you forward incrementally. If you are trying to improve your relationships by being a better listener, you might start with the practices of releasing a full breath before you respond to a question. Notice when you do this for a period of weeks until the pause becomes a habit. Follow-on steps can be then adopted in succession, such as using a stock interjection (e.g., 'I believe') before responding to conversational information. Take time with each step. Don't be impatient. You are making shifts in your routines and behaviours, not drastic changes.

You can spend as much time as is required to reach automatic improvement. During the process, ongoing dialogue with a carefully selected coach-monitor can:

- Remind you of your overarching desires when you question your choices.

- Call on your strengths when you question a goal's achievability.

- Celebrate wins with you, no matter how small, as significant steps in your journey.

- Mine the learning from each lapse so all actions are seen as valuable instead of setbacks.

Keep reminding your brain you can succeed so it will support you instead of protecting you. Transformation is more likely to stay on track if you make a point of noticing your accomplishments every day. When you accept that you must change a behaviour through habit conditioning, the act of letting go of old ways takes constant self-encouragement. It is easy to be discouraged. You might feel rejection and embarrassment if your attempts to change are rebuffed by others. You have to try out less than perfect behaviours. Asking for monitor's support and assistance can make you feel vulnerable, yet social support is important to help you override emotions that can trigger your brain to give up your motivation. Sharing your desires with others will strengthen your commitment.

Creating consistent quantifiable recorded evidence that you gradually succeed is invaluable and using a social support system that includes a coach or mentor can help become the happier person you want to be.

The habit–goal interface or interaction is constrained by the particular manner in which habits are learned and represented in memory. Specifically, the associative learning underlying habits is characterized by the slow, incremental accrual of information over time in procedural memory. Habits can either benefit or hurt the goals a person sets for themselves.

Goals influence habits by providing the initial outcome-oriented motivation for response repetition. In this sense, habits are often a trace of past goal pursuit. Although, when a habit forces one action, but a conscious goal pushes for another action, an oppositional context occurs. When the habit prevails over the conscious goal, a capture error has taken place.

Behaviour prediction is also derived from goals. An initial goal underlies a habit. The influence of goals on habits is what makes a habit different from other automatic processes in the mind.

Research Status

A recent study by Adriaanse et al. (2014) found that habits mediate the relationship between self-control and unhealthy snack consumption. The results of the study empirically demonstrate that high-self-control may influence the formation of habits and in turn affect behaviour. M. Reynolds (2018) asserts that on needn't plan progressive steps to realize a goal, in lieu suggesting creation of new habits.

Peter Dayan, at University College London (2017) demonstrates how we constantly update our goals through a dopamine-driven phenomenon called "reward prediction error". He is co-author of *Theoretical Neuroscience*, a textbook in computational and mathematical modeling of brain function. He is known for applying Bayesian methods from machine learning and artificial intelligence to understand neural function, and is particularly recognized for having related neurotransmitter levels to prediction errors and Bayesian uncertainties, Dayan has shown how our future behaviour is dictated by daily feedback on whether anticipated rewards and pleasures either fail to materialise or are more generous than anticipated. He maintains "Nature has endowed us with a fantastic system for optimising our behaviour," He is now working on applying the logic of decision making seen in the dopamine system to artificial intelligence algorithms. "That's how you get computers to make predictions." These developments have opened new avenues in the field of artificial intelligence as well as that of Clinical Psychiatry.

Advances in neuroscience signal benefits for patients with mental health challenges, and by extension to emotions such as happiness, euphoria and exhilaration. It demands brain work, and the brains sense-based interaction with a similarly complex environment. Dealing with such complexities necessitates powerful techniques. Computational psychiatry combines multiple levels and types of computation with multiple types of data in an effort to improve understanding, prediction and treatment of mental illness. This discipline, broadly defined, encompasses two complementary approaches:

- data driven and
- theory driven.

Data-driven approaches apply machine-learning methods to high-dimensional data to improve classification of disease, predict treatment outcomes or improve treatment selection. These approaches are generally agnostic as to the underlying mechanisms. Theory-driven approaches, in contrast, use models that instantiate prior knowledge of, or explicit hypotheses about, such mechanisms, possibly at multiple levels of analysis and most notably of abstraction. Researchers are reviewing recent advances in both approaches, with an emphasis on clinical applications, and highlight the utility of combining them.

Ray Dolan, of the Max Planck UCL Centre for Computational Psychiatry and Ageing in Berlin, Germany, has further explored the influence of dopamine on decision making, working from fundamental knowledge derived from decision neuroscience to study a range of psychiatric disorders, including depression, anxiety and obsessive-compulsive disorders, an approach encapsulated by computational psychiatry. As we age, people lose around 10 per cent of their dopamine-producing neurons, which can deplete a person's ability to predict future rewards accurately. Dolan has shown that this ability can be restored by giving older people extra supplies of dopamine. After the advances they have made in understanding rewards, researchers are now exploring how the brain responds to punishment. Dayan says the smart money is on another brain signaling chemical, serotonin. "That may be involved in punishment, but it's fairly speculative at the moment."

Conditioning

There are several processes involved in patterning and then conditioning (by repetition) of the nervous system: creating habitual psychological and physical behaviours. Given a fundamental understanding of these processes, stopping unnecessary patterns of behaviour (i.e. those arising in arbitrary, cultural conditioning, political and similar indoctrination, transient peer group pressure, socially engineered 'education', etc.) can be possible.

Ultimately, the generation of both unconditional interrupt (spontaneous physical negation by direct observation and action), and conditional interrupt (deliberate - based on pattern disruption techniques), depends upon 'doing' which is fostered by conscious expansion exercises and interrupt techniques that create doing by negation.

Pattern interruptions are designed to be carried out kinesthetically (i.e. by the physical body in direct self-awareness) - and not as mere word manipulations. Mere superficial reading, discussion or 'thinking about' a pattern or pattern interrupt as an intellectual behaviour merely perpetuates pattern continuity in the form of word: the description is not the described. The Body/Brain will interrupt destructive patterns - if allowed the opportunity to observe it directly (kinesthetically) - and intervene directly.

The individual needs to learn one or two key things with regard to 'conditioning' (which lies at the root of aberrant behaviour) - and then the rest is down to ingenuity in devising means of altering that conditioning - mainly by interruption, but sometimes by superseding - and implementing them.

An interrupt will normally work on its own. Proper interrupt will temporarily break the continuity of the behavioural loops that comprise an individual's' psychological conditioning or habit. Once the shallow levels of verbally driven continuity become derailed, then the underlying default - and benevolent/harmonious/wholistic biological - conditioning will kick in, provided the circumstances or associations that form part of the original condition are also addressed.

Pattern depends upon repetition and cannot exist without it. Repetition creates habit by patterning the form upon which on/in it repeats. Break the pattern and you break habit. Repetition of pattern, in whatever mode comprises vibration. Patterns exist as periodic oscillations, sometimes simple, sometimes complex - but even the most complex of oscillations can be broken into simple component parts (consider this as a Fourier analysis). Patterns do not exist only in mere 'words' and sounds, but in all manner of things - geometric pattern, colour, physical form, physical movements, rocks and crystals, architecture, science, mathematics, taste, texture, visual image, or fluid flow. Some are natural in that they occur spontaneously in nature, some, as culturally grown varieties.

Once you become aware of the fundamentals - by daily/moment to moment observation, not by mere intellectual discussion and theorisation - then you should be able to detect patterns in most things and in many cases deal with them as necessary 'on the wing'. Alternatively, you may use prescribed (usually tried and tested) 'techniques' as devised by others. The first method is best in terms of actual in-depth understanding; as for the second method, well note that somewhere, sometime, somebody devised that technique originally and perhaps you can improve on such general methods by devising some to suit your own particular circumstances.

'Patterning'

In 1879, Pavlov worked on the physiology of digestion, which culminated in his book, *"The Work of The Digestive Glands."*. During the course of his work, Pavlov noticed that salivation could be induced by the sight of food, or other stimuli that normally preceded feeding or in the association of some other stimulus with the feeding process. This led him to the discovery of the 'Conditional Reflex', now regarded as a fundamental aspect of learning and classical conditioning.

In a typical experiment, Pavlov showed that if the presentation of food to a dog was repeatedly accompanied by the sound of a bell, then the dog would come to respond to the bell as if it were food whether the food was presented or not. In other words, a non-natural response could be created by repetition and association of artificial stimulus and that the effect of the artificial stimulus persisted even when natural stimulus was removed. He measured the salivary response to paired presentations of food and bell and then measured salivation in response to presentation of the bell alone. He regarded salivation to the food as an "Unconditional Response," and the subsequent salivation to the bell alone as a "Conditional Response," because it is 'conditional' upon prior pairing between food and bell. He suggested that the cells of the 'Central-Nervous-System' changed structurally and chemically during conditioning. Pavlov's major work was translated into English as; *"Conditioned Reflexes: An Investigation of The Physiological Activity of The Cerebral Cortex"* (1927).

In his original experiments, Pavlov confined a hungry dog in a harness and presented small portions of food at regular intervals. When he signaled the delivery of food by ringing a bell, the behaviour of the dog towards the stimulus, (the bell), gradually changed. The animal began by orientating to the bell, licking its lips and salivating. When Pavlov recorded the salivation by placing a small tube in the salivary duct and collecting the saliva, he found that the amount of the saliva collected increased as the animal experienced more pairings between the sound of the bell, and food presentation. The patterning by presence of repetition of stimuli and pairing of a stimulus in a parallel pattern. Without repetition, the conditioning did not occur.

Speech in Conditioning

The manner in which we speak (and think - when thinking in words) actually conditions the structure of our nervous systems and physical forms and, accordingly, our perception of the world. It is not 'merely' a psychological process but rather a physical one in which the repetitive patterned sounds (or repeating electro-chemical sound images acting in the structure of the neuronic system in the case of verbalised thinking) actually condition the structure of that system. The word-form sound patterns we hear in speech (and which manifest internally, in imaging in the hearing sense, during verbalised thinking or internal dialogue) comprise a series of systematic complex grunts which were associated in our nervous systems, by repetition), to objective sensory experience in us as young children. We reinforced this by imitation - itself a form of repetition.

All this took place when we learned to speak - first in 'noun' (object), then adjective/noun, then verb, adverb and preposition/article/conjunction etc. as we became practiced in the rules of language. Children typically utter a first word at around ten months. At age one they have a 'vocabulary' (largely imitative) of four or so words, twentyish words at eighteen months and at age two something like two to three hundred. Somewhere between the ages of one and two years, the child actually 'understands', unconsciously but clearly, that language is a symbol system referring and describing the world around him/her; and becomes a 'member' of the conceptual world associated with the particular language system.

What is observed with your sensory apparatus is not the 'actual' or 'out there', but a reality filtered by the conditioning of the nervous system. It is filtered according to the conceptual base of your first learned language. Cultural similarities in the content of conditioning [culture in this context meaning the broad swath of human activities]. The biological, behavioural and especially linguistic will give rise to similar, or consensus, shared realities. The greater the similarity and intensity of conditioning, the greater the consensus.

Collective conditioned patterns - and their interaction with other patterned forms in the actuality of the unknowable, undifferentiated 'what is' - give rise to our nervous systems' view of the world, our differentiated reality. So long as we persist in those patterns, so long will that view persist. Shifting our cultural and linguistic patterns - the actual conditioning sounds - will shift our view of the world, which owing to the arrival of acrophonic alphabets, the printed word, standardised dictionaries, mass production, the workings of electronic mass media, the electronic computer and concordant languages - rapidly converges on a global scale.

The problems of the individual develop in what is commonly referred to as 'psychological conditioning' (but see above with regard to structural patterning of the nervous system) - the movement of human thinking processes - which occur primarily in language and visually based consciousness systems in the form of words and words describing fleeting. As the dominant species the behaviour of humankind - which comprise the fixated patterned behaviours of individuals - will significantly affect the short-term circumstances of all other life forms.

Repetition

It is a simple matter to distinguish potential dangers from many of the unconscious conditioned states: greed, desire, guilt, fear, jealousy, and indoctrination. The individual can act intelligently from moment to moment, negating them as they arise.

Since 'I' understand directly that excessive heat [e.g. a hot stove burner] can damage my body. I immediately withdraw my hand should it come in contact with any such hot object. This (intense) process occurs spontaneously, without any verbalised thinking, in any normally functioning person. From the immediate reaction to any direct contact that might occur, I acquire an element of (useful) psychological conditioning that keeps me wary of hot objects - I have, either by experience or education/instruction by others, a learned caution that such things are dangerous to me and, without any internal debate, repetitive looping in thinking processes or interminable weighing of pros and cons, I keep clear of them.

On these lines the body 'conditions' the psyche directly - and very few repetitions of intense pain/learning about hot objects are required. If we can observe the dangers of our psychological conditioning that arises through unnecessary acculturation and unconscious repetition - even in a relatively superficial way - and become aware of the processes and indications of its presence, we can naturally act and negate, instantly and effortlessly, in the same manner as we do in not placing a hand on a glowing stove burner. In the seeing arises the deep intelligence of the body as a reciprocal movement of reaching for consciousness expansion, and this will have done with any danger to its well-being instantaneously, effortlessly, as in moving away from the hot stove.

Carefully read [once] the following tale:

- Once upon a time there was a beautiful girl named Angel. Angel was the most beautiful girl in the kingdom. Angel was so beautiful that Prince John fell madly in love with her beautiful face. But Angel, who was incredibly beautiful, thought she was too beautiful even for the prince. So, Angel decided to join a rock band and be a backup dancer. The End.

You will recall the name of the protagonist Angel whose name is repeated six times, but less so Prince John who is 'mentioned' only once.

Advertising, Propaganda and Repetition

The effects of repetition on the public have been researched in detail for more than a century. The principal findings, with respect to advertising are as follows - and for the word 'advertising' below you can substitute: 'education', 'conditioning', 'propaganda', 'sound bite':

a. Repetition conditions the credibility to your claims in the subject (whether those claims are *credible* or not) and, if done properly, it will create a favourable attitude in the subject. The more exposure a person has, the more favourable his reaction to it becomes: brand recognition sets in. (but a limit to the number of repetitions exists).

b. Sequence and frequency of advertising influence the degree and duration of recall. Memory depends upon the cumulative effect of intensity of individual applications of stimulus and number of repetitions. (similar to weight training - weight x number of repetitions = muscle building effect).

c. Repeat advertising increases the chances the reader/listener/viewer will get exposed to it. This is fairly obvious, but there is more; to hit about 90% of the audience in a given 'channel' (TV station, publication, etc.) a repeat of eight times is needed (assuming 30 per cent of audience noticed it when it first appeared).

d. Interrupting ad campaigns brings about decline in the recall; persistence is important. When a message is no longer reinforced, people forget & the pattern is broken. Not only will patterned repetition 'increase your sales', but it will likewise burn ANY repeated image - sales, political, religious, propaganda, corporate, cliché, poem, word or other symbol - into the structure of your consciousness. Sufficient repetition will modify consciousness irrespective of whether the image happens to have any basis in fact or not, hence it is equally as possible to have memory that 'fairies are real' as it is to have memory of 'two plus two equals four,' even though the latter has basis in the commonplace (though not in quantum physics) and the other is without merit.

Once repeated images become entrenched; and they do so in the manner of habit - they will tend to repeat themselves when any associative stimulus occurs, much in the manner of Pavlov's dogs. Significantly, the stimulus does not have to arise in an external sensory source, an internally associated image (e.g. word) is sufficient to energise the implanted conditioning and give rise to streams of associatively linked 'internal dialogue' such that one eventually conditions oneself by internal repetition.

Images implanted into consciousness become implicit in the functioning of that consciousness; the nervous system alters materially to absorb them and they become part of it. Repetitions taking place in groups [and over extended time periods]. Another name for this process is mantric oscillation or mantric vibration. Plotted on an oscilloscope the constant repetition of any given word set appears as a periodic wave form.

Conditioning Methodologies

As individuals we were indoctrinated into our conditioning by the dominant culture in which we are born. From birth we had no means of resistance or comparison, we innocently accepted everything the extant culture fed to us irrespective of its practicality, relevance or otherwise. Our minds (the macroscopic structure of our nervous systems) were imprinted and deeply conditioned into our culture which, once implanted, exists implicitly and continuously in our conceptual frames. The continuity of that conditioning depends upon our continuing participation and self-energisation of it - and individual responsibility certainly lies here. If as individuals we can interrupt the conditioning, which means de-energisation of our (mainly unconscious) repetitive behaviours, then they transform.

The first step in this lies in observation. Observation is direct learning that brings these unconscious behaviours into awareness; only the individual can do this - but fortunately, help is at hand in the behaviour of other individuals, which is a bit easier to observe.

To put this into practice, for at least the next week attempt to be aware of the patterned behaviours in yourself and others and of patterns that surround you. In particular, and since as discussed in depth elsewhere on this page, repetition lies at the root of patterning so try to be aware of the repetition that goes on in and around you in the following 10 'reference points':

1. in speech, the use of words, tonalities and clichés
2. - mannerism
3. – dress
4. - diet
5. - repeated visual patterns
6. - time based behaviour (observing doings of self/others at set times)
7. - repeated sound patterns
8. - spatial behaviours (doings at set places)
9. - precision repeated physical shapes (mass produced objects)
10. - linear sequences of events (how one thing follows another in repeated sequence)

Perception of behaviours in others is generally the simplest view- starting with others and not by personal reflection if you would; but be sure to get around to observing yourself: the real learning by observation kicks in with the awakening of self-awareness. Try not to criticise, comment (indeed words - spoken or thought - will only get in the way and perpetuate the repetitions) or attempt to change any of these behaviours, just become aware of them at the outset.

The "Broken-Record"

One of the fundamental assertion techniques for getting your own way/self-programming/self-hypnosis is by deploying patterned repetition. The 'Broken record' method involves just that - emulating a record that has got stuck in a groove and goes around and around repeating the same thing irrespective of any objections or queries about what, how or why. It epitomises simple patterned conditioning of the mind of self and any others who might come within hearing range. The 'assertion trainers' recommend use of the technique when:

a) handling 'conflict' situations
b) saying no
c) clarifying questions
d) correcting superiors/those in authority
e) when expressing feeling or opinion and
f) in situations where (ironically) the 'other person' isn't listening

In using this technique, they advise the user to speak as a propagandist by stepping-through five points for each undertaking:

1. identify the point you want to make

2. make a short, clear statement of it (= a slogan)
3. stick to the point with no wavering, no explanation, variation or discussion
4. persistently repeat it, over and over again, ignoring any arguments, statements, questions or evidence to the contrary until you wear down and condition your 'audience' (and yourself...
5. use monotony such as to obtain near perfect repetition of the message

The supposed power of 'broken record' style lies in is its infuriating uniformity — a uniformity that eventually convinces even the most intransigent opponent (but note, owing to the 'self-conditioning' involved in the heavy repetition, it implicitly carries the seeds of self-delusion if the chosen slogan does not relate to some salient reality). It is also effective over time in that it supposedly develops the 'assertiveness' of the user over time. Additionally, if used continuously in relationship with another person it signals to the other that what the user says is not likely to shift irrespective of counter arguments. Both the previous statements are nominally accurate in that repetition fixates and hardens attitudes ('attitudes' actually comprising heavily fixated patterning of neuronic structure). The reality of the effectiveness of the technique actually lies, as the propagandists and advertisers have discovered, in progressively conditioning the nervous system by repetition.

The broken record technique is very often used by politicians, corporate executives and officials, in 'debate', and in individual and series' of speeches and interviews, wherein they will attempt to repeat a favourable (simplified = generalised & thus information deleting and misleading) slogan - nowadays known as a 'sound bite' - over and over such as to imprint the consciousness of listeners with misleading concepts.

Assertiveness trainers often make a big issue of the concept of 'rights'. The concept may stem from probably arising in the US cultural background of 'Bill of Rights', the United Nations Charter, civil rights movement and women's liberation. Typical rights statements, which the eager listeners are encouraged to repeat and hence implant (thus fixing 'attitudes' again), are as follows:
- I have the right to state my wants and set my own priorities.
  I have the right to defend myself.
  I have the right to behave independently.
  I have the right to express my feelings.
  I have the right to a fair reward for my work.
  I have the right to be treated with respect as an equal human being.
  I have the right to refuse responsibility for other's problems.
  I have the right to express my own opinions and values.
  I have the right to say 'yes' and 'no' for myself.
  I have the right to change my opinion.
  I have the right to reject poor service.
  etc., etc.,

Note the repetitive 'broken record' form associated with each individual statement (within the overall patterning of 'rights') of 'I have the right to...' and then note the gross repetition of the words 'I' and 'my' - which are sounds that neurotically pattern ego-image fixation and self-centred ideation. In a similar vein the same 'authorities' recommend the use of 'I' form statements as in: 'I don't like it when you_____. I want you to_____.' (we fill in the blanks with an emphasis on longevity goals).

Seniors Life Extension

'Broken record' is essentially self-hypnosis leading into automatic response of incantation of specific formulae in specific circumstances, but it is a self-hypnosis that gets projected, by repetition, into conditioning the nervous system of anyone who happens to come within range of it. The self-centred world views projected by broken record should not be allowed to pass unchallenged - otherwise, by persistence, they will become predominant. Hence dealing specifically with this problem - a problem which roots in conscious, selfish conditioned behaviour. The repetition of a simple pattern ad nauseum until that pattern becomes entrenched in the neuronic structure of the person using it and, in some circumstances, the people who hear it.

Negation Techniques

Many assertiveness training courses emphasise that their students should learn and develop "The *'Art'* of Saying No" and recommend that this be done by *practical repetitive conditioning* using the following (typical) techniques:

1. Role play.

   One if two partners repeatedly and calmly answer 'no' (out loud) to any questions the partner(s) ask, the questions often being prearranged by the course organisers. The idea here is to condition the student - using tens and tens of repetitions - to actually come out with the word 'no' as a semi-automatic response & in doing so overcome any pre-existing inhibition to saying 'no'. Unfortunately, as with a lot of this training, the questions do not arise from a general 'any type' of question ground but are usually 'I' related - and the recurring 'no' responses serve to fixate ego.

2. In-Public

   The student is encouraged to go into various shops, restaurants, bars & public places and ask strangers for various things, examine them and then say: 'No I don't want that' (or some similar mantra) without offering any explanation. If challenged/queried they reply in similar manner - being sure to say 'no' and using 'broken record'. Again, the idea is to get used to saying 'no' as a semi-automatic response. Again, this comprises an adaptation of the basic 'broken record' technique of monotonous repetition (of 'no') irrespective of question, person or circumstance.

The essence of 'assertiveness' lies in the repetitive fixation of consciousness around the ego. Many people learn to balance this this quite naturally in their childhood environment, but some - those who might have been conditioned to introversion at an early age - do not and are genuine candidates for corrective assertiveness training. Carried on excessively such 'assertiveness', owing to its fixation and disproportionate emphasis in consciousness on ego, in the form of 'I', 'me', 'mine. and 'my', can become selfishness and aggression.

Deliberate, as distinct from the more powerful and immediate 'negation' type body interrupts, are dealt with in depth towards the end of this page but as an interim measure, one technique for dealing with the pernicious, conscious 'broken record' behaviour is presented here.

Insofar as pure associative temporal (linearly patterned)

conditioning is concerned, it is possible to use any pattern - but broken record uses specific language patterns that attach themselves to the extant patterns in the body. As said before, these are normally associated with the 'i', 'me', 'my', etc. patterns.

Tailing

The principle used here in breaking up such patterns is to persistently add onto the tail of a pattern in various ways such that the pattern in the same way that 1234567 does not equal 123456789. Adding to a pattern (or subtracting or reversing etc.) creates a new pattern. The old pattern becomes subsumed in the new and thus gets 'derailed'.

Three practical means of achieving 'morphing' of broken record statements by adding on to tail end are possible:

1. *shifting/reversing sense (grammatical)* This is achieved by considering the original 'broken record' statement and finding an appropriate word fragment, word, or combination of words that will either shift, reverse or otherwise destroy the meaning of the statement.
2. *generalising/depotentiating (grammatical)* This works particularly well on 'Statements of Rights' type broken records but can be adapted to work equally well on most forms. Basically, what you do is allow the speaker to make his remark and then add to it the shift that: 'what applies for her/him also applies equally well for the rest of the world': i.e. (s)he is not unique and the broken record statement (s)he makes becomes modified to apply to the general case (thus depotentiating the 'ego' element).

3. *interrupt* This is potentially the most powerful form of pattern disruption by 'adding' on to tail ends in that, depending on the nature of the language fragments/patterns used, it will effectively derail the heavily fixated, looping thought processes of the speaker by causing temporal 'blank out' into 'Trans derivational search' (that 'at best' can last for tens of seconds or at worst will break the broken record with a 'what?') as they attempt to make meaningful sense of what is happening to them.

With all these techniques, you need to listen carefully to the broken record to establish the precise word form and meaning. Then you need to invent a word pattern to shift it (walk away and give yourself sufficient time and space to do this if needs be; the effect, once you introduce the shift, will be permanent and worth the consideration). You may phrase the shift in terms of the speaker's viewpoint or alternatively (and better) make it stand as a general consensus view. If you can make it humorous then so much the better. Once you have the new word element(s) then every time you hear the 'broken record' you must persistently add them to the tail end such as to create a new pattern and make sure the speaker hears it every time. Monotonously imitate their voice and pace delivery to make this all-the-more effective.

Doing this will gradually, and repeatedly, re-condition the speaker's consciousness to the new pattern - whilst simultaneously protecting you from the original broken record & conditioning yourself in the new statement. That's why you should choose it carefully & accordingly, either make the word element(s) match an accurate description of practical, consensus reality as much as you possibly can - or design them to make the statement humorous.

Examples:
- 'Your price is excessive: reduce it' *"if you agree"*
- 'Your president is not a crook' *"He is an incompetent"*
- 'The International Conglomerate' does not pollute the atmosphere' *"In Antarctica"*

As before, you add the same words/fragments monotonously every time they use the specific broken record pattern, giving as good than you get.

The essential process here is to add word fragments/patterns that *transform and de-energize* any grossly one-sided, selfish point of view.

In strict terms of pattern conditioning (and disruption) it is possible to additively associate anything with anything. Accordingly, the sound pattern that arises in: 'I am a wonderful being' can be morphed severely into: 'I am a wonderful being/banana disgusting watchstrap' which will cause (if repeated) scrambling & derailing of meaning in *any* linguistic sense. More mildly (but smoothly and subtly) it can be sonically morphed into: 'I am a wonderful being/"myself is fun".' This interrupts by pivoting around the word 'being' and creates a grammatically ill formed, ambiguous double-statement (that simultaneously creates confusion, destroys the concrete, fixated form of the original assertion and implants a new one of: 'being myself is fun'.

Two options are defined:

1. Pure disruption - by severe interrupt [e.g. humorous counterpoint] is indeed amusing to see the gaping mouth and blank stare of an 'asserter') or
2. Creative subtle, gentle forms. [e.g. the double statement]

For best confusion you should use not less than a two word 'tail' - the exception being when the broken record pattern being directed against you ends in an ambiguous word or phrase you might be able to apply a single word with great effect.

Become aware of how often, in fact, you normally need to repeat and rely on repetition of elements of your existing vocabulary and how it confines you within its limits and within the aural sub-limits of its phonemes. Acquire phonological awareness by doing and you will realise that not only do you write using these repetitive patterns, you also speak and think in them - and neutrally and physically condition your being as you do.

Memory, Physical and Psychological Acquisition
The 'past' does not exist except in the memory of individuals, in stored images of various kinds - visual, sound, taste, feeling, scent - in the cortex. Memory is usually accessed by energisation of the various stored image by word symbol, either spoken or generated in the mind as thinking which manifests as 'internal dialogue' in the sense of hearing.

Individual conscious memory is partial, incomplete and inaccurate and generally fades as the time period between experienced events and memorisation of them increases. Memory can be broadly divided into two principal types (although some overlap obviously occurs).

A first type of memory is 'physical': viz. how to walk, read, ride a bicycle, talk, swim, drive a car, write, manipulate tools, etc. These are learned by the body on a trial and error repetitive basis, often through feedback and imitation of others already adept in the specific field. These are 'learned' or more correctly 'acquired' in order to function in the physical world.

On the other hand, there exist memories evidenced principally in word and visual image - so called 'psychological' memories - which can be observed to fall essentially into two categories: practical and reminiscence.

Practical memories comprise things like knowing one's name and address, how to find one's way home, how to boil an egg, where to find food, remembering where one put one's shoes, being able to read a map, etc. etc. Each of us has a vast repertoire of these practical memories which we have usually learned by some process of repetition and imitation. They are unlike 'body' memories in that no great physical motor skill (kinaesthetic learning) relies on them. They often do depend upon some motor skills for their successful execution (e.g. changing a fuse requires tool use skill, knowing one's name and address relies on language.) Practical and physical memories generally arise on the basis of need or effortless desire.

Reminiscences are made up of primarily of visual and word images of the behaviour of the self (and others) in situations that have gone. They depend upon the energisation of the nervous structure, with the form of word and/or visual images - in reaction to (principally) - habitual, repeated word images for their existence. Some typical language patterns kinducing/predicating the energisation of reminiscence are:

- what if...
- can/do you remember...
- I remember...
- I/we used to...
- X used to...
- if only

- I shouldn't have...
- I could have...

The predicates are followed by word patterns that relate to events that happened in the past, a past that only exists in memory, in imagination. This exists as fact: the past is imagination. It does not exist anywhere else, and events that have gone cannot be changed by any amount of speculation, words (thought or spoken), worry, repetition or conjuring of visual images.

Once a train of thought or conversation (= joint, collaborative expressed thought) has been established by such predicates, the essential character of that train will be maintained by the use of past participles (tenses) of verbs; in most vernacular speech and thinking this means that significant repetition of the following words occurs:

- was
- were
- said
- went
- had
- did
- remember
- recall

The unnecessary diversion of attention and energy into reminiscence changes nothing - apart from diverting energy, attention and awareness from the present and mesmerising those temporarily involved in such conversation or thinking. [Inattentive thinking in internal dialogue, also known as 'down time', can usually be detected in others as it usually is accompanied by:

a) stillness in body - especially neck and head - or repetitive body motion, and

b) eye fixation - often taking the form of looking at nothing in particular or 'into space'

Reminiscence is generally inefficient of impractical, it doesn't change anything; it is an act of inattention based upon habitual repetition of certain language predicates that create trains of speculative (mainly word) images. An exception is in argumentation where the arguer is skillfully using and association of the hearer's reminiscence to connect to the argument 'positively'. However, these images themselves are partial, incomplete, inaccurately remembered and full of omission owing to the manner in which word symbols naturally delete information from that which they attempt to describe.

Word repetitions, either spoken, sung or in writing (which gets converted into internal dialogue in the reader) become parallel or compound; with visual and non-language aural associations. Likewise, the use of internal repetitions (in slogans) of music, rhyme, rhythm, alliteration etc. implants tonal associations and repetitions which act as mnemonics for the slogan and/or the product name.).

News and Fake News; Authority and Sourcing

It can be shown that something like 80% of the information that gets presented to the general public by the mass media as 'news' in fact originates from what might be broadly called 'authority' - central and local government, political parties, government departments, police, courts, medical, scientific and religious bodies and so on - across the broad swath of media which includes National and local TV, radio and press. (This figure is established for democratic countries; in nations with more authoritarian forms of government it is higher.) The majority of the remaining 20% of supposed 'news' mainly concerns celebrity, sport and other forms of entertainment and 'information' originating from corporate sources.

The reasons for this situation are complex - social engineering and spin by government and their agents, uncritical, lazy and compliant journalism, complicit self-censorship, editorial policies, various forms of propaganda and campaigning, the 'need' to keep owners/advertisers/sponsors happy, covering topics taken up by rivals, giving the public 'what they want', etc..

Over-stating particular viewpoints by means of repetition with the effect that supposed 'news' (most of which is not 'new', novel or contemporaneous) becomes nothing more than propaganda, the content of which is established by the originators, enabled and distributed, often unwittingly and/or uncritically, by print and electronic broadcasters, such as to condition and manipulate public perception.

What about slanting, fakery and cliché? Do you detect evidence of slanting of fact by means of adverb/adjective, stereotype and cliché? Are there any 'EVIL dictators' in there, 'drug BARONS', 'RAMPAGING lunatics', 'MAD geniuses, 'CHEATING celebrities' 'ABSOLUTE certainties' "GENUINE Antiques" and the like? What about the political news? Is the man with a gun 'an insurgent', 'a freedom fighter', 'an invader', 'a member of the coalition forces' or 'one of our brave boys'? What are the implied perceptual structures presented in the 'news' relating to objects, characters and events in the stories? Are they fair and genuine, or can you detect spin and prejudice?

Seniors Life Extension

Now, and this is the ultimate test in terms of validity, consider what practical use the information might be to you, and further, if it is actually 'news' (in terms of being valuable, informative and up to date) or whether it has degenerated into something else. The fact is that repetition conditions perception.

The 'news' you have appraised might be topical, or more rarely even useful, when attended to once a day, but beyond that, as your data should be demonstrating, it becomes nothing but organised, sophisticated and irrelevant propaganda that dulls the mind. Knowledge brings action - and you know where the off switch is.

R. Hesketh asserts: "In all fields of endeavour, repetition is one of the more powerful ways in which a community establishes its 'facts', but the facts thus established are often unsound. The scientific community is not immune."

The patterns which get repeated most (and particularly those that get repeated in an organized & regular fashion) become paramount in the conditioning of consciousness in both its collective (cultural) and individual forms; the whole exists as a function of the parts. 'Pattern', in the broad context, means any pattern - sonic, visual, kinaesthetic (physical body feeling), olfactory (scent) or gustatory (taste) that repeatedly impinges on and thus affects the human physical sensory/nervous as a whole the term includes internally generated imaging in the form of visualization, non-verbal sound imaging and internal dialogue. Pattern affects consciousness implicitly because consciousness comprises awareness channeling through pattern in creating form.

In the latter stages of the second millennium AD human

consciousness became increasingly focussed in language. This occurred primarily because of eleven innovations that prospered:

1. the advent of the printing press
2. the Industrial Revolution
3. widespread introduction of low-cost mass-production and mechanical drum printing
4. the parallel improvements in general wealth, health, standards of living, social and educational standards
5. political changes, particularly nation-states and apparent democratisation
6. telephony and telegraphy
7. consumerism, commercialism and attendant advertising
8. use of psychology and of propaganda
9. the unprecedented rise of mass media in the form of printed works, radio and television
10. mobile telephony
11. computers, search engines and social networking

As a result of these changes - occurring first of all in Western Europe but spreading ever more rapidly and cascading into other geographical areas and other cultures - an almost universal literacy has come about and with it an ever increasing dependency on, and focussing of attention in $_{LANGUAGED}$ thinking (arisng from both visual and spoken word input, and general commonality/consensus in that thinking by virtue of restricted vibratory symbol sets), and hence a restless, chattering, linguistically driven perception largely restricted within the confines of the particular language symbols.

Mankind has slowly lost its former innocence, tranquility and quietude of agrarian pre-monetary times. In return for undeniable material, the majority of humanity has lost the opportunity for quiet meditation, time to contemplate and freedom from the gross intrusion of the oscillating patterns we recognize as word. All gone, superseded by collective endless noise and chatter that impinge on the individual consciousness (which reciprocates by adding to the chaos in the collective consciousness) from all directions and increase with every day that passes as population grows and intensifies with number and packing density.

When a child becomes a member of the languaging group he/she develops the languaged 'I' image of ego), it becomes self-perpetuating owing to the associating nature of memory and its ability to connect the sounds of various vibratory grunt symbols not only with 'real' objects in an 'external' physical world but with the 'internal' store associative symbols and images that comprise language in memory. The reactive energization of this memory may occur by either external or internal stimulus in any given situation, but once set in motion internal stimulus perpetuates itself in the form of the almost endless and mainly useless noise of internal dialogue that fills the majority of the modern human being's waking hours.

As well as cliché, chant, slogan, jingle and 'motto'; poetry and music contain repetitive figurative vibratory elements that enable them to modify the consciousness of the listener by persistent excitation of neuron groups. The more a neuron group gets triggered by a particular signal, the more that signal modifies the group in its own image and thus obtains priority in memory.

Tonal "Clues" and Using Music/Poetry

When memory responds (the process which comprises the essence of 'thinking'); it responds preferentially in terms of the patterns that dominate the neural structure. Poetic and musical forms use various repetition (viz. low frequency forced oscillation) techniques to take hold of consciousness. Some of these comprise:

- direct repetition of complete sound forms (individual words, phrases, sentences)
- repetition of syllable and morpheme (through alliteration and rhyme)
- repetition of pitch
- timbral repetition
- rhythm

In certain forms - especially in songs that evoke strong emotional feelings (e.g. 'I will need you forever'.) - the implicit associative mantric repetition can actually condition powerful negative depressive states, 'song' being probably the most powerful mnemonic form known to mankind. Once conditioned, re-association (by the song, music or word) will re-evoke these states in 'anchor triggering'. This can also be turned in the opposite fashion; and put to beneficial use. If no 'emotional' form (or any other meaningful word form) has attachment to a complex word group, then such structured groups can be used as powerful mantric (vibratory) interrupts. Playing and re-playing positive music in relation to reward *expectation and* playing/replay discordant interrupting scores in connection with negative habituation are prime examples.

A 'poetic' mantra demonstrates a typical rhythmic 'verse' form with compound internal structure (the overall structure & internal repetitions and compare with popular song and poetry). We have developed:

Seniors Life Extension

> a) conditioning of the upper reaches of the nervous system occurs principally through repetition
> b) you are surrounded by repetition in all manner of patterned forms
> c) words are a particular form of sonic form and that the repetition of words - individual, in phrases and particularly in rhythmic alliterative and rhyme form (i.e. slogans, jingles and mottos) is used by those who wish to confine and direct attention in particular directions of their choosing

The objectives of those who might wish to condition you with their points of view are likely to be as diverse as those very points of view, but one thing is for sure and that is when you come across sonic repetition in speech - especially when it includes rhyme, alliteration and slogan/cliché - then the originator of such is attempting to condition your thinking processes and selectively programme your memory. Advertisers use these techniques (think of a particularly annoying jingle), as do religious and political propagandists, corporate and institutional bodies & their agents (some naively), and self-seeking manipulative individuals.

The Principles of Repetitive Conditioning

Obvious repetitive conditioning often occurs most commonly on six axes:

> a) in direct time sequence (repeating single words or syllables (e.g. Education, Education, Education)
>
> b) contiguously - in fragments - by the continual, but subtler non-continuous, repetition of particular words and phrases (as in 'Let's talk about Trump. Trump knows Everything you do, absolutely

Everything, and he keeps written records. you can be sure that Trump writes everything about you down in his book of records etc.,'. The effect of this kind of repetition is powerful and hypnotic in that it overloads and distorts the listener's perceptual processes by repeatedly, and deliberately, placing undue emphasis on specific words/concepts and directing attention towards them. When senses are stimulated then that very motion in the sensory apparatus creates the experience we name 'attention': repetitive stimulation narrows attention on itself.

c) by repetition of identical, word (and often time and tone) perfect messages/slogans/instructions periodically over extended time scales. These Word perfect, 'news' bulletins, official announcements and jingles in commercial breaks appear periodically (and not necessarily regularly) throughout a given time period.

d) in the repetition of cliché, slogan and motto occurs. These 'mantras' supposedly contain kernels of wisdom related to the topic being propagated but on closer inspection such 'wisdom' turns out to be meaningless drivel BUT a form of drivel that is very carefully structured rhythmically and tonally so that it is easy to remember, chant and roll easily of the tongue. Such repeating mantric form overwhelms and dulls the senses of the listener and speaker alike & ultimately causes the neurochemical patterning of the listener to resonate with that of the speaker such that the former absorbs the point of view. In extremis, this process (of narrowed repeating attention) resembles a hypnotic state. Examples of this type of mantric form are: 'Think

Drink Pink Gin' (rhyme and rhythm), 'Eine Volk, Eine Reich, Eine Fuhrer' (word repetition and rhythm) and (external and internal alliteration).

e) in emotionally ill-formed song lyrics, the extreme multiple repetitions of which dramatically exceed the normal constraints of everyday prose speech by means of presentation as 'song' (would you permit someone to come up to you in the street and whine: 'I can't live without her/him anymoOOoore...' at you twenty times? Such structures are common in 'song' (and song is arguably one of the most powerful mnemonics available to humans) and they perniciously invade and distort consciousness - particularly that of vulnerable teenagers - with emotional negativity since their thought processes eventually become entrained with these words.

f) By participation - and this is possibly the worst form. In the more pernicious forms of conditioning you will be invited to 'join in' the process by repetition of (speaker given) word forms and associated rituals of physical behaviour (which further reinforce the patterning). Think company song, parrot style 'learning', political slogan, hymn, prayer and religious ritual, football and protest chants, etc.

These illustrate some of the more obvious ways that repetition is used to manipulate human consciousness; there are other, far more subtle ways which you should be on the lookout for (for example the compounding of sonic and visual images) - but they will inevitably rely upon some form of repetition.

It can be asserted that through much of this, a trained

person can spot any attempts to condition you virtually immediately by revolting against them. You can act, either by:

- immediate interruption or contra-diction
- removing the source (see below)
- moving away from the influence of the source.

Significant exposure to the repetitive (hence oscillatory) inputs to the human nervous system indicated below will create disproportionate and generally harmful patterns of conditioning that in turn desensitise perception and awareness. Additionally, many of these behaviours are 'de-inviduating' (tend to take away individuality and render the subject a member of a crowd or group of various kinds) and are deliberately used by those who would seek to manipulate such groupings [e.g. senior citizens, religious affiliations, national alliances etc.].

The repetition of stimuli in the forms demonstrated - either in isolation or compound form - inevitably creates preferential islands and 'noise' in consciousness as it forms semi-permanent association patterns in the electro-neurochemistry of the nervous. Through extended repetition and exposure, repeated stimuli form themselves into elements that participate in the normal reference state of the nervous system as an implicit part of actual, perceptual and conceptual. In a modern non-ascetic society, it is impossible to entirely avoid the stimuli types indicated, but nevertheless a serious and alert observer will find it relatively easy to significantly reduce exposure either by bringing the activity to a halt or moving away from its source - and in doing so he/she will reduce radically the internal noise and obscuring agitation that such oscillations impart in the mind pool. The internal forces that sustain non-essential conditioning can be negated and thereby atrophy. In tandem, as this conditioning structure dissolves, then slowly, but certainly, a state of heightened sensitivity and alertness spontaneously arises - the awakening of intelligence.

The barrier to enhanced awareness and the essential nature of ignorance comprise one and the same thing - non-essential electro-neurochemical noise that has developed in parallel with, and in consequence of, mankind's linguistic split consciousness. The non-essential noise originates in unconscious, patterned oscillation (repetition) of elements of the physical body, oscillation that actually possesses energetic momentum. Once stilled, this comprises the ground of an unconditioned person.

You can avoid repetitive, external forced oscillation of your body and nervous system and subsequent vibrionic entrainment by:

    a) moving away from the vibrating source
    b) interrupting the source
    c) modifying the impacting pattern of the source
    d) non-participation with the forcing oscillation

Be aware that forcing repetitive oscillations come in all sensory modes (visual, aural, kinesthetic, taste and scent and combinations thereof), multiple forms, shapes, sizes and can comprise simple and compound frequencies ranging from UHF to ULF. Note that in the manner of the law of precession [previously discussed], and Newtonian physics which maintains that once a body (and that includes a human body) has been set in a state of periodic motion then it will persist in that state until compelled by an external oscillation to do otherwise.

Simply put; once you have acquired a habit (a state of conditioning) then it will stick until something occurs that unsticks it. Break pattern, break habit. You can best out-flank an unsavoury habit by not acquiring it in the first place. You will 'get into the habit' by repeating any action over and over again, and there are many actions which are antithetical to life extension. Citing a specific example: finishing each and every meal with a sweet for dessert is likely to upset any calorie reduction motivation which you intend to implement. Using repetition aurally [e.g. soothing or uplifting music as well as verbal cueing]to replace dessert [or some desserts] is a positive enforcement intended to establish suitable habituation; thereby converging with the newer 'positive goal', and thus hard-wire it into the reward system of the brain.

Nutrition for Life-extension

Ageing is fundamental to life-prolongation. We have already examined the mechanisms identified as age-related. This book is only a single source material for the reader's life-prolongation purposes, but it is tailored to the needs of those who have retired from conventional work assignments and have elected to extend their lives by taking concrete actions [including goal execution and habit alteration]. The best knowledge of nutritional and physiological sciences will provide tangible 'first' benefit. Further study, along with practical application of the recommendations set out here, will put you in the driver's seat.

Some of the practices described below, particularly the consumption of large quantities of certain nutrients for health improvement [and incipient life expectancy improvement] are innovative. If you choose to pursue them; you do so upon your own responsibility. No one should take 'major doses' of supplements or amino acids without consulting a physician *trained in nutrition*. Some people can be adversely affected by these, and particularly so among seniors who are prescribed medications (and often too many) for specific health concerns. Because of these potential complications, the approach to nutrition should always be informed. Properly applied, programmes have turned genetic limitations into talents and limited talents into successful applications. This book is intended to provide the necessary growth to match demands placed on the body by meeting improved body function head-on.

Be forewarned, you are daily bombarded by a mass of media nutrition/supplement 'facts', marketing bull-manure and boldfaced lies: all claiming to be the best in nutrition.

When celebrities, particularly when they are seduced by money, lend their names to fat and sugar loaded materials as 'official foods of their sport', trust goes out the window.

Unbiased information is left to us only in research presented in peer-reviewed scientific journals. These sources are 'dry' and difficult to navigate without specialised training. Though precise and accurate for the sciences provided, the study results rarely make it into popular media because they lack the luster of celebrity.

Old Time Nutrition Religion

It is often still maintained that nutrition has no magic to it, and that all the 'health consciousness' requires is a simple three-square-meals a day. selected from among four major food groups:

- Meats
- Dairy foods
- Fruits and vegetables
- Grains

This is a false folktale carefully crafted by the meat and dairy industries; and contradicts everything modern science has uncovered concerning human nutrition. To put it succinctly, putting meats and dairy foods on a par with other nutrients is one big reason why athletes in North America have not kept pace with the athletes from countries where science is more carefully attended. This book owes its foundation to the premise that many senior citizens who are required to participate in longevity sciences are not getting the truth about nutrition. The rest of the world has begun to leave English speakers behind.

Many seniors are warehoused in assisted living facilities where meals are provided as part of the 'pensioning-off' housing process. Portions are generally too small to meet the needs of anyone moving significantly – which is the third law of health improvement. It is also a truism that such room and board meal plans almost invariably provide a mix of constituents which are in conflict with 'optimal nutrition'. Those doing practically any 'work' must augment the food on offer to thrive, often passing up what is proffered at each meal-call. Therefore, the newly minted or continuing older longevist must fork out of his wages for proper nutrition – especially for nutritional supplements.

Anyone who follows the 'four food groups' condemns themselves to an inferior level of health improvement; perhaps so inferior that they will harm themselves by a continuation of physical exertion without optimal nutrition. Obsolete ideas concerning nutrition seek to persuade the individual that they are not in the mainstream of society science the field of nutritional biochemistry has recommended to the USDA that they abandoned the four food groups, reclassifying meats and dairy products is optional foods as early as 1991. Evidence that excessive intakes of those products in North America are strongly linked with high rates of cancer, heart disease, diabetes, obesity and osteoporosis; all of which senior longevists must minimize. Meat and dairy definitely do not improve bodily function in persons involved in heavy exertion.

Building Blocks for Longevity

Optimal body function, especially in those doing a programme of incrementally stepped exercise, who are always pushing the limits, cannot occur without daily ingestion of a precise mix of more than 50 substances. Some you need a lot, and some you need only infinitesimally small quantities. But they all are required in correct amounts. The first five are:

1. Oxygen
2. Hydrogen
3. Carbon,
4. Nitrogen
5. Sulphur

We need these in large quantities and they are widely contained in foods and in the air, we breathe, so supply is generally not a problem the remaining nutrients we need in medium or small amounts require less plentiful occurrence in our environment and maybe significantly deficient or absent entirely in any particular food that we consume. Among the elements that are required in medium amounts daily that our bodies demand:

1. Calcium
2. Phosphorous
3. Magnesium
4. Sodium
5. Potassium
6. Chloride

And minerals that are required in small amounts daily are:

1. Iron
2. Silicone
3. Iodine
4. Zinc
5. Cobalt
6. Fluoride
7. Arsenic
8. Boron
9. Copper

10. Chromium
11. Molybdenum
12. Manganese
13. Selenium
14. Nickel

We required vitamins for proper nutrition. Those specifically identified for our purposes here include:

1. A
2. B3
3. B-12
4. C
5. K
6. B1
7. B5
8. Folic acid
9. D
10. B2
11. B6
12. Biotin
13. E

What are called "co-factors" are also required:

1. Choline
2. Co-Enzyme Q 10
3. PQQ
4. Bioflavonoids

Among the most important building blocks are essential amino acids. These include:

1. Isoleucine
2. Phenylalanine
3. Leucine

4. Threoninelynine
5. Tryptophan
6. Methionine
7. Valine

Every single one of these identified elements are required; and they and interact with each other in precise synergy to produce, maintain, and renew the physical body. If even one is missing or in short supply then the functions of all the others are impaired. To adapt to proper nutrition initially, the first step is to grasp just how much you can be affected by what you put in your mouth.

Needs and Individuality

Biological biochemical individuality is now so well-established that recommended dietary allowance should be revamped on its ear. These values have been so long misused by medical practitioners and the food industry as a standard for individual nutrition that the error becomes nationally accepted and has given rise to numerous general recommendations that are supposed to fit everyone. They in fact benefit no one because these values never were meant to. For individuals the handbook for RDA states on it's first page: "recommended daily allowances are recommendations for average daily amounts of nutrients that population groups could consume over a period of time; they should not be confused with requirements for a specific individual". If you endeavour to employ RDAs for the purpose of nutrition you will never ever reach your life's potential. The RDAs were developed for average persons, who by cultural definition are sedentary – and those electing for better health performance are *not* sedentary.

Evolution developed the human to convert an ingested mix of certain compounds that convert nature into muscles, bones, organs, glands, and others. The human being is an interaction of nutrient compounds. Whenever you mess them up, they will mess with you. It is required to understand how much abuse of food intake disturbs the exquisite precision of nutrient use by the body. There are two examples to illustrate how this takes place:

- You require only a few micrograms of vitamin B-12 each day. Your blood contains only about five nano-grams (billionth of a gram per liter), less than a 'speck'. It represents less than 1 part-per-million of body weight; yet if you lack that amount - your whole-body declines, and serious disease takes hold as with pernicious anemia, which gradually destroys the sheathing which protects your nerves. This in turn leads to blindness, mental health challenges, and possibly death.
- A second example is iodine where 50 µg per day is considered sufficient for most people. This amounts to a quantity so tiny that you could not see it with the naked eye. However, a few molecules of iodine occur in different foods and are broken down and transported straight to the thyroid gland if they are available. There they convert to an inert chemical from which powerful thyroid hormones are created. These control your energy supply, mood and even how well your cognitive functions perform.

The same applies to all of micronutrients and forms a mystery to research science as to just how such minute amounts and substances hold keys to health, society and life itself. But they do so. When we coax vehicles to perform adequately we are very careful what we put into them; yet we put some totally wrong fuels into our bodies without concern.

Synergy

Synergy of nutrients is the first principle of modern nutritional prolongation sciences. Nutrients operate only in multiple interactions with each other. Case studies which only consider how an individual vitamin, amino-acid or mineral perform in the human body are worthless. By way of example; vitamin D in the human body plays a controlling role in the metabolism of calcium and phosphorus. The B vitamins work only in synergy with each other. The list of established first level interactions between nutrients increases every year with the change in approach to consider these complex multiple connections have been established for many vitamins and minerals vitamin E interacts with copper to influence protective membranes subject to damage by free radicals (stress oxidation). When vitamin D is deficient, or zinc is used by the body to pinch-hit for the missing nutrient, this action has the added effect of increasing body levels of copper. Unfortunately, many healthcare providers and the general public still operate under the erroneous concept of single nutrient information - it is multiple interactions of nutrients is the basis of our biological functioning and it is only in the last 30 years that research has been able to key on this interaction.

Because of the principles and synergy deficiencies also affect other nutrients B2 deficiency impairs B-12 metabolism, which impairs formic acid metabolism. Folic acid dysfunction and then affects vitamin C metabolism the resultant depletion of the body from of that vitamin impairs iron absorption impaired iron absorption in turn encourage excessive copper absorption which then impairs zinc metabolism. These, in paired functions, did not make endurance exercisers really ill or even stop them from working-out. The performance was way below expectations. Individually designed nutrition programmes, adequate in all nutrients which permit the synergetic interaction to take place, can restore anyone setting out toward long life to good health.

Biochemical Individuality

Individually design nutrition programmes lead to a second principle of nutrition: biochemical individuality. Because of genetic variations, individual bodies are biochemically different from each other. Some people have narrower feet than one another, or high arched feet, or flat feet - the range of individual differences in foot configuration is enormous. Making one size of shoe to fit everyone would be patent ignorance. Yet that is exactly what happens in most 'nutrition programmes.

Health food stores promote dozens of different brands of one-size-fits-all supplements as if they were exactly what the individual body requires. You don't have to do complex tests to know just how wrong they are - look at your peers. Body differences radically occur between all people, from the shape of your nose and toes to the texture of hair and the range of movement of limbs required for exertion. Insight is just as different muscles, glands, organs, nerves, and the brain differ from one person to the next. For optimal performance the body requires different nutrition from one person to another. To be effective a works programme of nutrition has to fit individual forms and functions at least as well as your shoes fit your feet.

Biochemical individuality is well-established in medical science. Roger Williams began to patiently document the huge difference in individual needs for nutrients more than 50 years ago. He showed that, for optimal growth, animals require 20 times the vitamin C when compared one to another. The difference in bodily unit usage of vitamin A varies up to 40-fold between individuals [and accordingly it's replacement need is a multiplicand]. Unique differences in nutrient requirements are now established for a variety of vitamins, minerals, and amino acids. Excretion of vitamin C is a normal function that helps protect the urinary tract. Increases in excretion rates are often used to measure at what level in the body tissues become saturated with the vitamin the excess spills into the urine and can be measured. The amount that stays in the body gives the saturation level. A number of research studies have indicated some people could take 5000 mg of vitamin C and show only a little increase in excretion all our vitamin C was being used by their bodies. Other people showed a large increase in excretion of vitamin C after taking only 1000 mg it was found that biochemical individuality in the use of vitamin C is at least tenfold if anyone tells you otherwise don't believe them. Ask them why they can't all wear one size shoe.

Life-Style and Health Extension

It would be easy to design individual nutrition programmes if biochemical individuality alone determined personal need. Unfortunately, lifestyle and environment radically affect the needs as well. Nutritional requirements vary with lifestyle dynamics such as food quality, smoking, alcohol, pollution (water and air), medication, competitive demands, training for exertion, age and many other factors.

Decline in hematological red blood status which determines your capacity to use oxygen effectively is a common problem. It can be reasonably assessed by measuring blood levels of three variables hemoglobin the red pigment that carries oxygen, the proportion of blood composition of red blood cells, and red blood cell count (RBC) which measures the number of red blood cells in the blood.

In a study of 12 male marathon participants who doubled usual training distances to an 8.5-minute mile showed large reductions in hemoglobin from 'excellent criteria' after 20 days; realizing at that time passage only marginally 'acceptable levels. Their usual nutrition was unable to maintain the blood components essential to carry oxygen to their tissues.

The principal nutrients involved in making red blood cells are iron, zinc, Folic Acid, vitamin B6, vitamin B12, and vitamin C. When individuals' nutritional intake levels of these nutrients were studied over the 12-week period of increased training level - they maintained their red blood status and increased their maximum amount of oxygen used and improved their performance.

The essential lesson from this study is that individual lifestyle demand dynamics shown with changes in sustained exertion, drinking alcoholic beverages polluted water, work medications for other purposes and of variety of variables radically affected nutritional need. Unless your nutrition programme is matched to your lifestyle, you cannot expect optimal performance in heavy work.

Precision in Nutrition

The most common objection to the need for individual nutritional programmes matched to biochemical individuality and lifestyle is:' why can't a One-A-Day vitamin pill with a megadose of all nutrients sort out what needs to be done, and excrete the excess'? To do so violates the principle of precision. Each individual has a particular range of intake of each nutrient that will yield optimal function. Below that range function becomes sub-optimal because of toxicity. To optimize for health-work, you need a programme that puts all of your nutrition in the optimal range.

Taking arbitrary megadoses of nutrients into the toxic range as many do, disrupts performance in four ways:

- Some vitamins and minerals are toxic at only 10 times the recommended daily allowance the toxic dose of vitamin A for example is 25,000 international units One-A-Day vitamins commonly contain 10,000 international units. A handful of these pills would subject you to sub-clinical vitamin A poisoning. The same applies to selenium, chromium, fluoride, iron, and vitamin K.

- The interaction between nutrients changes radically when some of them are taken to excess; essential fatty acids deplete the body of vitamin E, and zinc interferes with iron metabolism and disrupts copper metabolism.

- Megadoses of nutrients determined by guess-work are not correct ratios to each other. Vitamin B6 has to be present in adequate amounts for the body to absorb B12. Many other essential interactions require nutrients to be the in the correct ratios to each other for optimal function to occur, and issues of biochemical individuality.

- Individuals vary in their needs for nutrients in ways that cannot be covered by megadoses, not only because of individual genetics but also because of activity, rest cycles and lifestyle. A person who exerts regularly, for example, has increased requirements for certain of nutrients such as vitamin E and chromium - but not for others. A person who lives in a small polluted area has increased requirement for provitamin A and other antioxidants that would be an overdose for people living in clean air environments. There are hundreds of such factors determining nutritional needs that cannot be covered by arbitrary dosing. The only answer is an individually designed personal nutrition programme.

Physiology of Nutrition

A first principle of nutrition is physiological dynamics. Unlike drugs, nutrients do not have rapid effects. There is no quick fix. The business of nutrition is to build a body that can perform better. Blood cells last 60 to 120 days; in 3 to 4 months your whole blood supply is completely replaced. In six months, all of the proteins in your body die and are replaced, even the DNA of your genes. After one year all your bones and even the enamel of your teeth is replaced - constructed entirely out of the nutrients that you consume.

The time course is well identified by the course of deficiency diseases. Removal of all vitamin C from a diet over four weeks causes blood vitamin C to drop to zero. No symptoms of disease are seen at four weeks. You have to wait until enough of the healthy cells have been replaced by unhealthy cells after passage of another 12 weeks before symptoms of scurvy start to damage the body. When you implement an optimal nutrition, programme don't expect rapid results.

In a research study active people supplemented to try and improve their hemoglobin, hypocretin and red blood cell count; but after one month of supplementation there was no improvement at all. After six months, however, all three markers were significantly improved. This is the reason the athletes are almost always required to execute a minimum six-month programme of nutritional supplementation before improvement results (or deficits) are observed.

One size does not fit everyone!

Initializing a Programme

Fluids

Both the muscles and the brain, which are responsible for performance, are more than three-quarters water. The lungs which intake oxygen are practically 90% water. The most important nutrient in your body is water. The quality of tissues, performance, and resistance to injury is absolutely dependent on the quality and quantity of water consumed by exercise in temperate conditions employees 2 L of water a day in breath, sweat, and urine. Stressful lifting requires over 8 L of water a day for heavy work. A 75 kg person is a composed of 50 L of water which is replaced every six days.

The type of beverage must be considered. These are all mainly water and include commonly milk, fruit juices, coffee, soups, and even fruits and vegetables. Dehydrating muscle by only 3% will result in an approximate 10% loss in strength, and an 8% loss of speed. Performance grinds to a halt. - and the long-term benefits of an exertion programme are impaired.

Common limits for tap-water maximums are reflected in current European Union standards:

- Acrylamide 0.10 pg/l
- Antimony 5.0 µg/l
- Arsenic 10 µg/l
- Benzene 1.0 µg/l
- Benzo(a)pyrene 0.010 µg/l
- Boron 1.0 mg/l
- Bromate 10 µg/l
- Cadmium 5.0 µg/l
- Chromium 50 µg/l
- Copper 2.0 mg/l
- Cyanide 50 µg/l
- 1,2-dichloroethane 3.0 µg/l
- Epichlorohydrin 0.10 µg/l
- Fluoride 1.5 mg/l
- Lead 10 µg/l
- Mercury 1.0 µg/l
- Nickel 20 µg/l
- Nitrate 50 mg/l
- Nitrite 0.50 mg/l
- Pesticides 0.10 µg/l
- Pesticides - Total 0.50 µg/l
- Polycyclic aromatic hydrocarbons 0.10 µg/l (Sum of concentrations of specified compounds)
- Selenium 10 µg/l
- Tetrachloroethene and Trichloroethene 10 µg/l (Sum of concentrations of specified parameters)
- Trihalomethanes — Total 100 µg/l (Sum of concentrations of specified compounds)

- Vinyl chloride 0.50 µg/l

While working to enhance (improve) raw water from their sources, municipal jurisdictions are limited by time and money and, though well-meaning, they reduce the prescribed maximums as closely as possible to the maximum allowable for economy. This, unfortunately, is not adequate for performance purposes. We will outline the impact of water authorities meddling with aluminum salts in the text below.

Water 'Improvement'

For optimal performance an unbreakable rule is to continually consume the required quantities of water for performance. It is important to consider whether the water that you intend to consume maybe polluted. Even at 500 ppm of contaminants some studies have indicated even groundwater is dramatically polluted. It has been estimated that there are more than 60,000 chemical contaminants possibly existing in water we consume. Municipal water supplies likely harbour at least 1000. Water authorities do what they can, through sedimentation filtration chemical conditioning and disinfection by chlorine. Toxic metals, pesticides, industrial contaminants are still there when it comes out of the tap. In addition, carcinogens from chlorine itself occur. These are responsible for disabilities of the liver and cancers. Bottled water is a North American Goldmine; with up to 425 indigenous brands marketed. Imports account for approximately 35 brands. This industry is unfortunately still self-regulated.

Be aware that most bottled water is simply tap-water put through an additional minimum conditioning's circumstance by filtration. This makes it taste better and that's why it's profitable. What is euphemistically called 'Springwater' is from a spring but is usually just tap-water from that source. Distilled water is the only clean bottled source. Virtually everything is removed from the water by steam distillation. Accordingly, they contain 2 to 12 ppm of contaminants, which is about as clean as you're going to be able to realize.

Due to the costs and uncertainties associated with bottled water, many people are cleaning the faucet water at home. Boiling water on its own only affects organisms which are shown to induce illness. Simple filtration generally treats only particles larger than 5 μ. Four step osmotic systems may remove up to 97% of contaminants. This translates to 22-40 ppm contamination. Steam distillation in the home is by far and away the method of choice. Keep in mind that pure water does not cause the chain of minerals from the body on absorption in the intestine, the mixture immediately blends with body fluids and becomes part of you. The lack of minerals from steam distillation do not cause health issues. You get your minerals from proper nutrition. Plant minerals provide the main source of minerals to animals and most members of the human race.

The bottom line is steam distill water which you intend to consume. Most available systems are capable of producing the required amount of water for family consumption, but certainly for consumption by those who are going to engage in heavy labour.

Dehydration and Rehydration

Whenever the body is robbed water, performance during exertion is compromised. The biggest three factors involved are:

1. overheating,
2. disruption of chemical balances,
3. dehydration.

The most important of these is overheating.

Exertion increases body temperature in proportion. The body tries to maintain a resting temperature of 37°C by removing extra heat to the skin via blood. It dissipates into the air through evaporation of sweat. Blood must also carry oxygen and nutrients to the muscles and remove waste from the muscle through metabolism. Throughout these tasks the central feature is blood. The higher core temperature rises, the more blood is used for cooling, and the less is available for muscle activity. So, the cooler you stay during exertion, short of being cold, the more muscles are able to perform.

Outside of the range between 35 and 36.8°C, the body will always sacrifice muscles that are functioning – placing emphasis on simple temperature regulation because a decline in muscle function occurs, even to the point of complete immobility - and may be life-threatening. If body core temperature rises by as little as 5°C, normal biochemistry ceases and the individual is fatally affected.

Exertion and Fluid Demand

Heavy exertion increases heat production in muscles to more than 20 times their resting rate. Even at optimal hydration rates and in cool environments this heat load can raise your core temperature by 5° within 15 minutes. When the temperature rises above 42°C your physiology searches temperature reduction. A large volume of blood is shunted to the skin for emergency cooling, causing blood pressure and cardiac output to tank, depriving muscles of oxygen. The usual simple symptoms are those of overheating in the face, throbbing in the temples, and a chill over the chest and trunk. People at heavy labour, pressed for performance, will push core temperature upwards to unsuitable levels. This produces dizziness, weakness, and disorientation and frequently the risk of heat stroke.

One purpose of this book is to inhibit age decline in capacity to carry out enduring activity that begins generally after age 35. This can be done with the right nutrition and training, but the individual must stay cool and to keep body temperature below 38.5°C. Air temperature and humidity at the time of exertion are important and experienced individuals praise overcast skies and mist or light rainfall. The rule of thumb is that external temperatures and humidity of 22° and 70% respectively are optimal. Do everything to stay cool. Drink all fluids as cold as you can personally take them, to give a reservoir of cold in the core. Warm up, but only just enough to break a light sweat. Wear light coloured clothing, and as unencumbered as possible.

Stay out of direct sunlight. Expose all the skin possible to maximize heat loss through evaporation of sweat. Wearing clothing that 'wicks away sweat' is a minimally effective. Even the best 'wicking' sports shirt creates a clammy human environment over every square centimeter that it covers. Contact humidity kills evaporation. There are times that a mesh shirt is required by sun exposure, but operate in as little clothing as possible, working without any shirt would be advisable if Sun is not an issue.

The American College of Sports Medicine recommends that the individual not enter into activity when the ambient air temperature exceeds 28°C. Unfortunately, the weather doesn't always cooperate; but even in hot conditions if you follow the cooling rules and also maintain hydration, body temperature usually plateaus below 39°C. If dehydration occurs temperatures jump sharply - and again blood is diverted to the skin for emergency cooling. Muscles and brains are left short of oxygen which is carried by the blood. Energy metabolism also shifts and starts rapidly consuming the store of glycogen. To avoid overheating and sustain performance you must drink enough water to sweat significantly.

Many people often object that they don't feel thirsty during exertion. This is true, and sensors in the throat and gut are inhibited during strenuous exercise, even though you are losing water rapidly. Do not be fooled by lack of thirst; any exertion beyond five minutes of duration requires effort to remain hydrated.

The first step to maintain hydration is to work up carbohydrate consumption for a period of not less than six days before heavy exertion is commenced. It's beneficial that they are also a great source of water after digestion, Carbohydrates are converted to glycogen and stored in the muscle and liver for use as fuel. In order to store a single gram of glycogen the body has to store 2.7 g of water. Careful carbohydrate loading can double your usual glycogen store when the metabolism of glycogen during exertion takes place.

The second step is pre-hydration. Pre-exercise loading yields lower performance temperatures and smaller weight losses. Drink extra water for two days before undertaking dramatically increase exertion, then between four hours and one hour before activity drink 250 mils every 10 to 15 minutes. Consume another 500 mL between 30 and 20 minutes before activity. Make certain to urinate. Drink nothing during the 20 minutes before you start the activity because your stomach requires that much time to nearly empty (otherwise you start with a lot of water washing about, which is uncomfortable and may result in cramps or inhibit breathing during heavy exertion). The kidneys almost shut down urine production entirely. Practice this during training for heavy exertion to determine the capacity to water load suitably.

The amount of extra water you retain from drinking extra for two days before exertion varies widely from individual to individual, and with the amount of sodium and other nutrients consumed in the diet. With water loading and carbohydrate loading you have a sufficient reservoir for sweating during exertion and to be optimal you must use every millilitre.

It is essential to drink during the course of exertion. It has been shown with the athletes that temperature rise to 39°C at comparable level can be maintained throughout exertion with hydration. With out adequate hydration temperatures continue to rise after 60 minutes to uncomfortable levels and end in unsuitable performance, and possible heatstroke. Even if you are water loaded before exercise, you should take all of the plain water that you can. During any long exertions, in most circumstances, take 200 mL at every stopping point possible. It is desirable to finish exertion with a less than one kilo less mass; and keep body weight loss below 2%.

Drinking water is easy. Getting the body to absorb it optimally may not be. Cold water below 10°C is absorbed faster than room temperature water. It supplies a reservoir of cold in the stomach and would absorb considerable body sheet do not gulp water. Gulping swallows air which disturbs stomach function and slows absorption. The same applies to carbonated drinks. The gas slows absorption. Avoid them.

The use of pure water is highly recommended. It is absorbed rapidly. With particles it is absorbed more slowly. This include sugars. In addition, dissolved particulates make it harder for water to pass from the stomach to the small intestine where it is absorbed.

Accordingly, commercial drinks which contain glucose or sucrose or simple sugars should not be used, as they inhibit absorption. The absorption decrease is approximately 12% of the value achieved through plain water absorption. Not all sugar is however bad. Fructose at 2% enhances stomach emptying and preferentially restores glycogen. Similarly, polymerized glucose, that made by chaining simple glucoses, allows for rapid and introducing that material up to 5% actually appears preferential. Combining fructose with chained glucose in a ratio of 2 to 5% has been demonstrated to be effective.

After you have exerted, how do you get your back to normal? The most important thing is to be rehydrated. Your stomach is in a highly acid condition after work and almost empty. Your muscles are loaded with debris of metabolism. Your glycogen reserves are depleted and, you are in electrolyte overload because of the percentage of body water lost is always greater than the percentage of body minerals lost.

Rehydrate immediately by drinking plain cold water. Sip don't gulp. This requires effort because the first response is still inhibited after performance. Avoid juices especially citric juices which contain acid and high sugar contents. Until you have consumed 1.2 L of cold water. Avoid carbonated drinks, beer, fruit, yogurt, chocolate bars, muffins, and all other sugary fatty compounds. If your stomach is generally sensitive; a quarter teaspoon of bicarbonate of soda can be consumed or two capsules of buffering compound supplement can be beneficial. Do not sit down or lie down after heavy exertion no matter how tough this may be. Muscle cramps and injuries often occur because of insufficient blood getting to fatigued muscles – particularly large leg groups after running or accelerated walking. Much of the force for blood circulation comes not from a heart but from working muscles. Keep drinking and walking if possible.

Continue drinking for at least the next 12 hours if practicable. A common problem with endurance work is chronic partial dehydration. This is especially important for individuals who are going to work the next day in similar high stress environments. Where working the body is required repeating times remember that the urination system in your body will assist you in establishing baselines.

Carbohydrates

Carbohydrates are equally as important as are fluids - to replace muscle glycogen quickly. After 1.2 L of water, eat any easily digested complex carbohydrates such as whole grain pasta, oatmeal or optimised breakfast cereals.

Soil Degradation and Food

Since the end of the Second World War the prevalence of nitrate phosphate potassium fertilizers has been employed by as much as 97% of North American farms. In order to make a living, this economic system has replaced mulching, manuring and crop rotation. Our body's system requires selenium, chromium, calcium, magnesium, iron, copper, iron, molybdenum, zinc, cobalt, boron, and vanadium and other trace elements. Our bodies cannot make these minerals and they must come from nutrients derived in the soil and/or by supplementation. They are not in the produce produced by NPP farming. Without consuming every one of the essential minerals in adequate quantities no one can expect top performance in heavy exertion. From the soils we have today and the produce and food animals that grow upon them; this becomes a practically impossible task.

Preparation and Storage of Foods

Soil degradation is only the first of several problems in our food chain. Further nutrients are lost in ripening, storing, drying, cooking, freezing, blanching, pasteurization, hydrogen nation, ultrathin Thracian and multiple other processes of food production. The recommended daily allowance handbook states the vitamin E content of food varies greatly depending on processing, storage and preparation periods during which large losses occur. Vitamins C can be considerably lower because of the destruction by heat and these processes also affect vitamin B6. 50 to 70% is lost in processing meats and 50% or more lost in milling cereals. Folic acid may be destroyed up to 50% during a household preparation, food processing and storage there. More than 80% of magnesium is lost by removal of the germ and outer layers of the cereal grain in the practice of enriching flowers. Freezing of meats can destroy up to 50% of vitamin and riboflavin, and 70% of pantheonic acid. Modern food processing has stripped our food of many of its vitamins.

Now we also have irradiated foods that do not rot and maybe years old and devoid of vitamins by the time you get them to eat. Genetically altered foodstuffs (GMO) have altered mineral and vitamin content in ways not yet understood. There are four mechanisms to offset produce degradation: buy your produce close to where it comes from, (e.g. farmers markets), buy only an organic vegetables and fruits straight from the health food store, buy at a local farm outlet, and buy only certified organic produce.

Fuel in Nutrition

The type and amount of carbohydrates employed to provide the right fuel mix, and the timing of their intake, establishes an optimum supply for any performance in endurance exercisers. It is demonstrated that carbohydrates are a limiting fuel since no matter how lean individuals are, they have fat calories to spare. The body employs some fat during extended activity, depending on the biochemical individuality, blood oxygen levels, blood free fatty acid levels, and conditioning. With Carbohydrates, however, you can run out quickly. A caveat on fat. Despite its high caloric content at nine calories per gram, in muscles, fat burns very slowly for energy. Primary fuel for exercise is adenosine triphosphate. It's a lot easier for the body to break down muscle glycogen and blood glucose into ATP than to break down fat. Consequently, ATP is formed of a lot faster from carbohydrates than from fat the rate of synthesis from carbs is 1.0 mol per minute from fats and the rate is only .5 mol per minute from fats. Accordingly, carbs yield twice as much energy as fats. During anaerobic exercise, which only uses carbs as fuel, energy formation jumps five times the energy level that can be realized from fat sources. Carbohydrates form the highest energy fuel of the three basic nutrients.

The effect of forcing the body to employ faster fuel is well-established. If exhaustion of muscle glycogen and blood glucose are at low levels, the body burns predominantly fats. Performance declines were radical. Endurance exercisers should design their carbohydrate nutrition so that they burn as little fat as possible.

Meat, Fish and Fat

Fat is a principal constituent of meat. The impression that beef, veal and pork are healthy and low in fat is fallacious. The public has reacted by seeing a decrease of some 25% in the consumption of beef since 1976.

It is common that the fat content of average trimmed pork exceeds 53%. If you value your health and longevity, fat content alone is enough to turn you off meats; but that's only the beginning. Most meats marketed in North America are seriously contaminated with antibiotics, hormones, pesticides and other residues. In 1991, in 90% of market swine and all veal calves, 60% of cattle, and 95% of all poultry; antibiotics have ben routinely added to their feed. The routine use of penicillin and tetracycline derivatives in animal feed has caused the inclusion of drug-resistant strains of bacteria which now remain in the meat you consume. Food poisoning bacteria kill thousands of North Americans every year and make 6 million sicker than acceptable. At least half of all chicken and eggs are contaminated. Free range organically grown meat that is chemical free and low-fat is hard to obtain economically. It is impossible to produce low-fat meat stock that are free of antibiotics, hormones and pesticides while remaining cost competitive against mass-produced livestock. Suitable livestock must forage. To secure free range status, organically grown meat is required to range on ground that which is chemical free. In return for the production on such land you find that the material is 25% leaner in fact.

There has been a widespread reliance on fish as an alternate to ground-based meats. Reports as early as 1992 have shown that 40% of the samples were beginning to deteriorate or spoil at the time of purchase the CDC report the fish and shellfish cause about 10% of all outbreaks of food poisoning in North America but maybe dramatically underreported. Fresh fish has virtually no odour. As soon as it begins to spoil it produces a chemical called trimethylamine which gives off a 'fishy odour'. This is a sign of spoilage. If tuna is to be consumed, make it skipjack or albacore. These are lower on the food chain because of their size, and only slightly polluted. Flounder and sole are the least polluted as is Australasian Orange Roughy. These are shown to be low in fat and contamination limited.

Foodstuffs for Longevity

For best health performance food is focal. The basis for optimum performance is whole grains and vegetables. These are good sources of carbohydrates. The same is true of fruits with the exception of their high content of simple sugars in many cases contain added sugars. In this context the best protein sources (more than 20%) are:

- Soybeans
- Split peas
- Kidney beans
- Dried whole peas
- Wheat germ
- Lima beans
- Black-eyed peas

- Lentils
- Black beans
- Navy beans

The best carbohydrate sources containing more than 70% carbohydrate include:

- Brown Rice
- Whole barley
- Whole buckwheat
- Whole rye
- Millet
- Wild rice
- Whole corn
- Whole wheat
- Rolled oats

The quality of food protein must be assessed by its content of essential amino acids, the ratio of these amino acids to each other, and their bioavailability the biggest problem of being and soy of product protein is taste. Because of predilection due to acculturation many people cannot easily convert bean and soybean protein sources because of undigested sugars which ferment in the gut with dramatic results. One product marketed as 'Beano' contains an enzyme which digests the errant sugars for you. It also works for those who suffer the effects from raw broccoli cabbage falafel, oat bran, whole wheat or other whole grains which are gas producing as a result of their sugar content.

Fibre

If you base your diet on grains and vegetables you will naturally get a large dollop of fibre. It does a lot more than the popular belief that it keeps one regular as digestion goes but, it holds down cholesterol and prevents colon cancer. Fibre is essential to reduce body fat and to stabilize blood sugar. Many authorities recommend that a high-endurance longevist get 40 g of fiber daily. It is not that simple; loosely defined fibre is not a food for humans, it is a part of plant foods that the human system cannot digest. The six basic categories are:

1. cellulose,
2. hemicellulose,
3. gums,
4. mucilage,
5. pectins, and
6. lignins.

To ensure best results you are required to consume some of each of the soluble fibres, including pectin as occurring in apples and carrots - and gummy fibre with oat bran. Insoluble cellulose as in wheat bran, and other grains are required. As with all foods, variety is required for proper nutrition.

Use food rather than that medical fibre preparations such as psyllium for best variety of fibers by cereals. Get the plain kind and buy un-sugared dried fruits separately to mix with them. Do this yourself as the fruits mixed into most breakfast cereals compounded for marketability for are unsuitable. Review labeling on breads in spite of the 'whole wheat' labelling. These lists cannot mix in favour of marketability. Avoid enriched flour. That means that the flour has most of the nutrients removed and a few added back again. It is unfortunately true that you get what you pay for, and 'proper' bread is always more expensive in the store than the mass-produced white bread offerings.

Air 'Quality'

Air pollution is a massive problem in most North Americans cities. In 35% of them, over 98% of individuals are affected. Substances that enter their bodies include; man-made chemicals, particulate matter and toxic gases all of which contribute to poor performance. What you breathe as polluted air last year affects your body today. Discolouration of air is primarily due of the result of industrial nitric oxide. This reacts with sunlight to form the brownish toxic gas nitrogen dioxide. The accompanying haze includes ozone as a result of car exhausts and the action of sunlight on nitrogen dioxide. And man-made hydrocarbons are also introduced that contribute. The worst is an unseen danger - carbon monoxide from the burning of fossil fuels. It is tasteless odorless colorless and deadly. No amount of good diet and training for heavy exertion can come by these pollutants in your air. You cannot develop suitable potential for work

The ozone layer above the earth protects us from solar ultraviolet radiation. Man-made chlorofluorocarbons are depleting this and making holes in an increasing the radiation poisoning of the plant. This layer 20 km above us protects us in an important way ozone. It also kills bacteria in food processing. At ground level the ozone layer's concentration would kill you in less than a minute. At a level of old .3 ppm in air, Ozone inflames human lungs, even while resting. Those expending a high effort take in 20 times the air of sedentary individuals. Lung damage to athletes occurs at less than .2 ppm. This is only one sixth of the value defined as clean air. In Los Angeles close to 200 days per year the ozone concentration exceeds this limit. No one operating in heavy exertion can tolerate such an exposure.

Seniors Life Extension

A principle programming problem with ozone is the inflammation of the bronchioles much like the inflammation which occurs in asthma. Breathing becomes inhibited and the energy costs of each breath increases consequently the maximum amount of oxygen the individual can take in is reduced modern scholarship is indicated that major cities suffer up to a 10% reduction in performance. The acute effects of ozone non-performance are only the minor problems. The continuing damage done to the body will prevent you from achieving life prolonging physical health particularly to brain, muscle and lung tissues. Ozone damages tissue by generating free radical chain reactions, damaging bronchioles of the lungs by attacking poly unsaturated lipids in cell membranes and damaging and killing of red blood cells by generating hydrogen peroxide with in the blood. The long-term effects can hurt potential performance for weeks or even affects that last a lifetime.

The human body had very little exposure to carbon monoxide during ancient times. In developing a system to extract oxygen from the air it could not also develop a system to exclude carbon monoxide. Blood circulating through the bronchioles of the lungs is required for human woven in the cells to absorb oxygen from the air and dispose of carbon dioxide weights. Newly oxygenated blood then reaches muscles and organs this is the way it should work but the red oxygen-carrying pigment in your blood has 210 times greater affinity for Carbon monoxide than for oxygen when a molecule of carbon monoxide and a molecule of oxygen compete for attention at attachment to hemoglobin the monoxide wins every time. In air polluted with carbon monoxide, the blood will pick up all of this pollutant. In the presence of monoxide less oxygen is available for work by both the muscles and the brain. This results in a loss of conditioning. Maximal oxygen uptake is reduced and performance declines. In blood, carbon monoxide forms a toxic compound called carbohemoglobin which is carried to the muscles, and damages everything it comes in contact with. Unfortunately, the body does not notice this. This feature is one that leads to car exhaust suicides being popular.

In this text we are not going to deal with the smoking of tobacco, which contains alarming chemical damage-causing constituents – but contains very high CO levels as well. Studies have shown that for maximal oxygen uptake in sedentary non-smoking individuals the reduction of maximal oxygen uptake on the order of 2.6% is very common. For those involved in heavy exertion this level is practically doubled. Compounded by smoking the effects are disastrous. Do not take a smoke-break.

North Americans are breathing unsafe air during the periods of smog and following a smoggy day. Those that live in rural settings, largely related to ground topography which traps pollutions and fosters inversions which may contain pollutants generated thousands of kilometres away and trap them smack-on-the ground. The immune system is weakened by inhalation of smog constituents. While efforts have been made by immunologists to identify environmental pollutants those causing immune damage have largely been unchecked, and in many cases have increased in recent years. The incidence of asthma rose by 58% in one 18-year period. There is increased risk of death as a direct result of air pollution. Obviously, longevists who are involved in a high endurance activity are breathing more heavily than the average public - and are subject to even greater immunological irritants.

Air pollution is affecting all metropolitan centres, and many small municipal settings. Toxic doses of these pollutants are occurring even when sleeping, depending on the inflow of polluted air. Health performance and life expectancy is permanently reduced. The first and most obvious strategy to be employed would be to take yourself out of areas at risk. Unlike contaminated food and water, there is no simple solution to the contaminated air you elect to live with. You cannot run and you cannot hide.

Any air cleaning device in the home is a reasonable option, and electrostatic precipitation plate devices are preferred when the air is polluted.

Urban-Suburban Settings and Manufacturing Centres

If life demands that you live and work in high endurance settings in urban area, a few safety precautions may prove invaluable:

1. Never work out during smog alerts unless you do so in a contained purified air environment

2. Never work out during rush hours when vehicle emissions pool due to congestion (morning and evening)

3. Avoid smokers and tobacco smoke environments

4. Run or Walk in traffic free environments

5. Work outdoors early in the morning before pollution counts rise

6. Avoid underpasses, orchards and areas of close tall buildings as these attracts and concentrate pollutants.

7. Work out with a mask when particulate counts are high

The major defense against air pollution is nutrient antioxidation. Most pollutants cause their damage through these mechanisms. Studies on laboratory mammals exposed to very low doses (0.1 ppm) of ozone in the air demonstrated that, in the absence of supplementation, lung lesions developed within two weeks. Those that received large doses of vitamin E remained (80%) healthy throughout measurement.

Because of the principle of synergy previously identified, vitamin E alone is unlikely to provide optimum antioxidant protection. It is recommended that all longevists exposed to such pollutants use multiple antioxidants.

Pollutant Exposures

We have touched upon water pollution and toxic gases in the air environment. These are, however, not the only pollutants that affect those in the high endurance activities. North Americans are exposed to toxic chemicals at home and in the workplace. Most companies do not publicize the possible damage to health caused by their products and processes. Urban pollutants rarely make you ill straightaway. Instead, they accumulate in bodies over long periods, progressively disrupting the functions of it. Usually they remain undiscovered until the full extent of disease is identified symptomatically.

'Legal levels' of pollutants may be orders of magnitude greater than those that will cause long-term damage. Even with chemicals that are well controlled, risk is not eliminated. Workers in vinyl plastics industries have 200 times more liver cancer than the general population.

Mercury poisoning is a dramatic problem. Mercury poisoning can be cured if caught early. Detoxifier's include vitamin E and selenium. Canned food has been shown to contain lead. It has been materially shown even in small amounts to cause fatigue depression and memory loss. This is the lead to the food and drug administration progressively lowering limits for lead in foods. They now consider that there is no safe level of lead. Thousands of sources exist and high endurance activities such as work involved motor coordination and balance which are adversely affected by lead. Avoid leaded gasoline, canned foods, blended paints, pewter-ware, and most cosmetics. Adequate intakes of zinc, iron, calcium, and phosphorus reduce the absorption of lead. Vitamin D works well too as a detoxifier of lead that is already present within your body.

Aluminum has been shown to produce toxic effects on brains and bones and should be removed from the food chain. Inappropriate levels of aluminum are found in the destroyed brains of victims of Alzheimer's disease. They weaken and embrittle bones as well. Heavy activity requires that bones support the muscle system. No one planning a long life can afford weak bones. Aluminum salts are used routinely in water treatment, particularly during summer months in massive quantities. To eliminate this risk don't drink water unless you distillate. Distillation is the correct term: filters don't remove these materials. Read labels for the words aluminum or alum: avoid these products, including aspirins that are buffered, underarm deodorants and anything which may contain them. Similarly, avoid slow cooking or marinating foods in aluminum kitchenware.

Don't work with these products; and shun them when they are involved in food processing and storage.

Seniors Life Extension

Limits on Exertion

It's required to have an individual monitoring system for signs of overreaching that tell you to back off and increase rest.

There are five basic quantifiers which allow us to determine whether our systems are overloaded:

1. walking heart rate
2. waking heart rate,
3. waking up body weight,
4. insomnia,
5. immunity.

The first sign of difficulty is demonstrated by the waking heart rate begins the day before you get out of bed by taking your pulse immediately on waking and recording it do it before you get out of bed. It is less perceptive when emotions, activity, food consumption, type of food, caffeine and alcohol affect the heart rate later in your day. If your waking pulse on any single day is elevated more than 8 bpm above its average level during a preceding week you are falling into a state of overreaching your abilities.

The second sign is waking body weight. The weekly average weight should not vary more than 1 kg even if you are frantically working. Most persons at hard labour see only a 5 kg variation during the course of a year. If your weight drops by more than 1.3 kg on any day from a preceding stable body weight - you are also falling into overreaching.

The third sign is insomnia. Nighttime is a time of rest because the adrenal cortical phytic hormones adrenaline and noradrenalin generated by activity interfere with normal sleep the rule is if you work at night yet suffer from restlessness, inability to fall asleep or too early awakening - you are falling into a state of overreaching. You may also experience abnormal mood swings during waking hours and a loss of motivation.

The last is invaluable, if you can access it. It is the immune function as measured by the complete body blood count. This is part of the usual blood screening. If you show elevated counts of segmented neutrophils, but impose sites, monocytes, or a combination of elevated counts of these immune cells and no infection or illness is identified, then you are overreaching. You cannot resolve overreaching by simply increasing sleep of programme of one-week remediation is called for:

1. Stop the exertion routine entirely for one week, then undertake light training that does not consume more than 30 minutes per day

2. Reduce protein intake to 15% of total calories consumed

3. Increase carbohydrate intake to 70% of total calories using predominantly complex carbohydrates with a low glycemic index

4. Increase antioxidants to 200% of their usual intake

5. Increase sleep to nine hours

Monitor the signs and back off work and increase your sleep at the first symptoms of distress. Rest and sleep are essential for nutrition to do the work required to succeed at hard labour

Dealing Down Fats

In some early scholarship it was recommended that the total intake of fats in the diet should not exceed 30% of daily calories as a target, with saturated fats less than 10% of the calories. These figures were proposed as a national standard more than 40 years ago. The body can use many types of fat as its largest source of energy they provide approximately 9 Cal of energy per gram. An endurance exerciser who presents 15% body fat carries 12% as an energy reserve. The other 3% is essentially body fat that acts as insulation and cushioning for vital organs. The 12% energy reserve for a 75 kg individual participating at hard labour for considerable period of time retains his store of 75,000 cal. That is much more than he will ever need for his activities. Compare this with sugar in the form of glycogen the body's other main energy source. In the same person his wife 450 g of glycogen reserve at 4 Cal per gram are worth only 1800 Cal because of the body cycle of glycogen use with exercise, and because of the obligatory minimum level of glycogen for muscles to function at all, there is only enough for limited work. So, the limiting energy source for exercise is always sugar, never fat. Most of the energy reserves are simply deadweight and inhibit performance. Longevists gain no benefit from eating fats above minimum thresholds.

Food fats and oils are composed of fatty acids. A fatty acid consists of the fact in a bit of acid chemical makeup is a carbon chain made of carbon and hydrogen atoms. Different fatty acids have different length chains short chain and fatty acids such as butyrate acid from butter have four carbons. Fish oil and long-chain fats that comprise most of the human brain have 20 to 24 carbons.

Saturated fat has all their carbon atoms saturated with hydrogen atoms; that is, they will not hold any more hydrogen. Unsaturated fats have empty bonds where hydrogen atoms are missing. These spaces linked up with molecules of other substances in the body, thereby making unsaturated fats much more biologically active. Saturated fats have no empty wings and are virtually inert. Their only biological role is as calories to be burned for energy. Since most endurance exercisers carry more energy reserves of fat than they will ever use, they have no need for saturated fats at all. They are difficult to avoid in our fat laden food supply and cannot be practically avoided. But to achieve optimum performance through nutrition you should make every effort to eliminated saturated fats the diet. Individuals at hard labour do require special fats, as the major components of cell membranes, around every soul and the body. These fatty acids are also used in exclusive ways in the brain, inner ear, eyes adrenal glands and sex organs. These are very active tissues and the special fats are essential for high level of oxygen news and energy transformation required for optimal performance. Without them the individual quickly succumbs and dies. When there is a deficient supply, optimum performance is impossible

The body has the ability to use all true long-chain fats more than 16 carbons in unsaturated forms, and to lengthen already unsaturated fats; by inserting empty spaces called double bonds. Through this ability it can make almost all the myriad of different fats it needs but there are essential fatty acids you cannot make, including linoleic acid, long-chain 18 carbons fats. They have to be provided by the diet; and form the only central fats essential to the individual.

Fish and Vegetable Sourced Oils

Three fat sources are considered; fish oils, EPA and DHA. The body itself also produces EPA and DHA in brain cells, the inner ear and adrenals as well as sex glands and other highly active tissues. These are made in the body from alpha-linoleic acid. In a garden-variety diet you don't get sufficient quantities through the degraded food supply; the body can use them from fish sources.

Be cautious of where the fish come from. The best sources of EPA and DHA are the high fat cold water fish: salmon, sardines, mackerel, and trout. Sole and flounder contain insignificant amounts. Clams, oysters, and scallops contain high proportions of EPA and DHA in their fats, but only small total amounts. The suspicion of contamination of these sources is substantive. If you use fish oils to obtain required EPA and DHA then there is no need to seek these out. You can use extra-virgin olive oil in cooking and salads. It is a good source of linoleic acid, the first essential fatty acid.

Extra-virgin olive oil is recommended. It is a high source of mono-unsaturated fatty acids. Studies have shown it has beneficial effects on the lowering of serum cholesterol and on blood lipids. It is the most palatable and easy to use of the good vegetable oils. Make sure is extra-virgin which by law describes unprocessed oil. If available seek out organic sources of extra-virgin olive oil. For the longevist for it is recommended that Borage seed oil supplement be taken.

The best vegetable source of linoleic and other sought for acids is flax or linseed oil. This oil has been markets available freely for 'food use' for a considerable period of time. Other sources of the two essential fatty acids are pumpkin seeds, walnuts and soybeans. The dark green leaves of leaf vegetables also contain small amounts. The fat preferences are as follows

Good oils

1. flaxseed – linseed
2. pumpkin seed
3. soybean
4. Walnut
5. Canola

Second Best:

1. almond
2. Virgin olive
3. Safflower
4. Sunflower
5. Corn
6. Sesame
7. Rice bran

Unsuitable:

1. Peanut
2. Cottonseed

Prohibited:

1. Palm
2. Palm kernel
3. Coconut

Canola oil was illegal until the mid-1980s but is now approved for use. This oil has very healthy levels of linoleic acid. Canadian produced canola does not contain significant quantities of Erucic acid to make it unsuitable.

Seek out un-processed oils. Modern processing changes the chemical character of the fatty acids in oils so that the human body can no longer use them. All nutritionally important fats are in what is called a cis chemical configuration that is, the hydrogen atoms in the carbons are all on the same side of the molecule because of their slight electrical charge, the hydrogen atoms repel one another and then the carbon chain these bins are essential shapes that make it possible for the special biological functions of the fats to take place.

The enemies of oils are hydrogenation, bleaching and deodorizing. These procedures are applied to almost all mass-produced fats and oils today. They changed the healthy cis configuration into unhealthy trans configuration. Processing rotates the hydrogen atoms so on opposite sides of the fat molecule so the molecule straightens out its curvature becoming essentially straight and loses its ability to perform the biological functions required by the body.

Virtually no trans fatty acids occur in nature. However. oil products used in cooking oils, margarines, fats used in breads, cookies, candles, chocolates, frozen dinners, pies, processed meats and other cooked foods contain high levels of nutritionally damaging trans-fatty acids.

Total fat requirements for hard labourers are considerably lower than the target 30% of calories recommended in the past. Take time to estimate the best intake. Some researchers indicated that 9 to 12% of calories from fat are suitable for the highly active. In comparison of national diets' those of the Japanese have a diet of 15% of fats and achieve low rates of degenerative diseases. The lower fat diet results in a lowering of serum cholesterol and a reduction in the amount of fats you have to carry in your blood.

Body Fat

Body fat is a stronger predictor of performance related to fats. Every ounce of extra body fat increases body temperature during exercise, not only because of the extra weight insulation, but also because there is less water available for cooling body. Fat is only 50% water whereas muscle is 75% water. Except for essential fatty acids, the only fat you should eat is that which you cannot avoid - keeping the fat intake below 15% of daily calorie intake is optimal.

In a common 3000 Cal diet this amounts to only 450 Cal that is 50 g of fat about 20 g will be unavoidable saturated fat and that leaves you 2 tablespoons of olive oil and flax oil or maybe a pat of butter on your toast. Add two meals of cold-water fish per week plus a daily capsule of gamma linoleic acid (GLA), and you are doing all we know about fats to improve performance.

Keeping fat intake below 15% is a difficult task. Milk is highly touted. 250 mL of whole milk is 87% water 3.8% fat (69 Cal) and 8% carbohydrates and protein (64 Cal). That makes it more than 50% fat (69/69+64). Don't drink it. Even 2% milk is over 25% Using the 9 Cal per gram benchmark and rounding to 10; Adding a zero to the fat content gives an approximate caloric value of fat. Divide the total calories per serving of food always given on the label. Take into account that more than 1/5 of the total calories are indicated by this rule - leave it on the shelf.

In ranking the fat content of high protein foods, the following distribution is recommended:

Recommended; Less than 5% fat

1. Cod
2. Sole
3. Flounder
4. Lobster
5. Crab
6. Muscles
7. Scallops
8. 1% Cottage cheese
9. Turkey breast

Those with 5 to 20% fat

1. Shrimp
2. Tuna
3. Chicken breast
4. Buffalo steaks
5. Sardines
6. Herring
7. Salmon
8. lamb or veal
9. Ricotta cheese

Those to avoid, containing 30 to 60% fat

1. Hamburger
2. Pork roast
3. Bologna
4. Frankfurters
5. Beef roast
6. Bacon
7. Steak, T-bone
8. Pork sausage
9. Cheddar cheese
10. Cream cheese

The complaint is raised by many that avoidance of fats can only be achieved through the consumption of sawdust-like foods in the diet. This is patently untrue because variety can be obtained from simple study at the market source.

The minimum requirements for the longevist in the arena of fats can be summarized by five parameters:

1. Eliminate saturated fats from the diet

2. Use extra-virgin olive oil as your main source of fat

3. Eat two meals weekly of cold-water fish (salmon, sardines, mackerel, and trout)

4. Take a daily capsule of gamma linolenic acid (GLA normally in Borage Oil)

5. Keep fat intake down to 15% of total calories

It will be worth while to do so for performance sake.

Timing Carbohydrate Ingestion

Divide carbohydrates into three categories:

1. Carbs before activity

2. Carbs during activity

3. Carbs after activity

There are controlled studies which show that taking carbohydrates during exercise enables endurance performers to postpone fatigue and perform at the highest level. It is required, if the loading of carbohydrates is to take place, during the endurance performance that glycogen muscle content be optimized. Basic biochemistry identifies that carbohydrates taken between exertion sessions have to be more important than those taken during that activity. Glucose in the blood from carbohydrates just digested cannot be used by the muscles nearly as effectively as muscle glycogen from carbohydrates taken some hours before. Unlike muscle glycogen which can be used directly for energy, blood glucose first has to go through a chemical conversion of the glucose by adding phosphate. This conversion is done by an enzyme called hexokinase. Hexokinase is a limiting step in the body's use of glucose. This material in human muscle has only low levels of activity. The biochemical limitation keeps the maximum use of blood glucose for energy much lower than the maximum use of multicultural glycogen for energy. The level of glycogen in the muscles before you start activity is the most important fuel determinant of endurance.

Designing a carbohydrate nutrition programme, the primary goal should be at to achieve the highest levels of muscle glycogen between the finish of one session of activity and the start of next. To do this begin eating carbohydrates immediately after you finish a session. It has been demonstrated that muscle glycogen synthesis after exercise occurs in two phases:

1. A very rapid rate of utilisation for about 4 to 6 hours

2. A much lower rate for the next 24 hours

The most rapid rate of glycogen synthesis takes place after exercise because of the low level of glycogen remaining in the muscles, which stimulates activity of an enzyme called glycogen synthesis that controls the glycogen storage. It's required to consume carbohydrates when glycogen synthase is really active. The amount of carbohydrates is also important. It has been demonstrated that the maximum rate of synthesis in the first four hours after activity occurs by feeding glucose polymers on the order of 225 g. Above that threshold no further effect is demonstrated.

Glucose polymers are complex carbohydrates made by extending glucose molecules so that they are more slowly digested and simple sugars. Maltodextrin as in wide use in foods for more than 50 years. It is a reasonable source of glucose polymers. It must be easily digested to cause fewer problems of gastric distress as occurs with the consumption of energy bars containing bananas and dates.

Complex carbohydrates are not the whole story. Immediately after intense exercise you need sugar quickly, to take advantage of the high levels of activity of the glycol's storage enzymes. Take sugar in addition to glucose polymers. Endurance exercisers often avoid glucose because they believe the simple sugar will be detrimental due to an 'insulin burst'. If the muscles have a high demand or glycogen replacement the glucose is shunted into muscles so fast that no insulin instability can take place. Fructose also helps. It predominately replaces hepatic glycogen as we recommend: take 225 g of liquid complex carbohydrates, glucose and fructose immediately after activities.

For the whole period of glycogen repletion and before a next bout of activity an intake of 650 g of carbohydrates per day is recommended by widely circulated research.

The actual amount different individuals, but varies widely depending on:

1. biochemical individuality,
2. activity intensity,
3. activity duration and
4. preparation.

Ranges of need, depending on individual applications, according to work type may be as high as twice the 650-gram base-line. Because of individuality, the overall guide should always be the individuals body fat level there is a tendency towards overfeeding for two reasons. First - a small daily insufficiency of carbohydrates is not noticed by healthy individuals. But over weeks of activity it leads inevitably to progressive exhaustion of glycogen stores, setting the individual up for overwork-syndrome. Second, and most importantly, slight [beneficial] overfeeding of carbs reduces the use of muscle protein for fuel and therefore spares the vital muscle tissue.

For an individual weighing between 80 and 100 kg and involved in heavy activity for five hours recommended a carb-load of 900-1100 g per day is expected. Eat carbohydrates in small meals throughout the day. That is because; to maintain glycogen synthesis you have to maintain a steady state of carbohydrates across the intestinal wall if that flow is interrupted for even a couple of hours in a 24-hour cycle after heavy activity through endurance work, and then because the glycogen storage is reduced. This reduction occurs because the activity of the storage enzyme glycogen synthase is dependent on a steady flow of insulin.

Simple sugars cause insulin fluid fluctuations that inhibit glycogen synthesis activity and reduce glycogen storage.

Slowly digested carbohydrates, that is those with a low glycemic index, cause much slower rises and falls in blood glucose and insulin level than' sugars. The basic problem that endurance exercisers face is to identify these fully digested carbs from an array of every day marketed foods. The glycemic index which was developed by Dr. David Jenkins provides the best approach. Simplifying recommendations for longevists to eat less or eat more of a food, the following glycemic index values should be considered:

High glycemic index foods to avoid:

- Glucose glycemic index 100
- Honey glycemic index 87
- Parsnips glycemic index 98
- Carrots glycemic index 90
- White potatoes glycemic index 70
- Bananas glycemic index 65
- Raisins glycemic index 68
- White flowered spaghetti glycemic index 56
- Cornflakes glycemic index 85
- White rice glycemic index 70
- White flour pancakes glycemic index 66
- White bread glycemic index 76

Preferred foodstuffs:

- Fructose glycemic index 20
- Soybeans glycemic index 15
- Kidney beans glycemic index 30
- Lentils glycemic index 25
- Sweet potatoes glycemic index 48
- Apples glycemic index 36
- Oranges glycemic index 40

- Whole-wheat spaghetti glycemic index 40
- Oats glycemic index 48
- Brown rice glycemic index 60
- Buckwheat pancakes glycemic index 45
- Whole-wheat bread glycemic index 64

It is not wise to take high levels of fructose just because of its low glycemic index and that it does not indicate sharp fluctuations in blood glucose or insulin. High fructose diets cause of rise in blood fats and a rise in blood uric acid levels. Both are degenerative conditions which longevists should avoid. Some is reasonable, too much about paying fructose is metabolized in the liver and yields greater repletion of the liver glycogen than does glucose if added to glycogen repletion drinks without seeking additional fructose and other foods sufficient voting is possible. Use glycogen repletion drinks that are predominantly glucose polymers but also contained some fructose.

Study what you 'prefer' against its on-line revealed glycemic index and pare-away the undesirables.

During exertion the glycogen content of muscles always decreases. Muscle glycogen is the highest energy fuel, better than liver glycogen, much better than blood glucose and far away superior to fats as is already demonstrated. As the level of muscle glycogen declines, the level of performance declines as well. Having muscles full of glycogen at the start of activity is the ideal state. There is no way you can fully compensate for suboptimal levels of muscle glycogen by taking carbohydrates during activity.

In a study of athletes involved in endurance, consumption of between 40 and 45% of daily calories from carbohydrates sources has been shown to be optimal. For endurance activity, taking carbohydrates during activity maybe the only way to maintain performance. It will never be the best performance, because bodies cannot use blood glucose as effectively as muscle glycogen. It is best to keep your muscles full of glycogen. In the final stage of the long periods of endurance activity liver glucose in blood glucose from the digestion of carbs taken during the activity can provide 90% of the carbohydrate energy. Resting muscle glycogen levels in the range of 100 to 120 mmol per kilogram are typical for individuals who are consuming sufficient carbohydrates for optimal performance. For high levels of activity glycogen levels of 180 mmol per kilogram showed fatigue and insufficient muscle glycogen after just two hours of its exertion.

When to take carbohydrates? It is essential to take the first carbohydrates three hours before exertion. Costill and others have shown that complex carbs taken 3 to 4 hours before exercise raised blood glucose in performance. It is recommended to habitually take 100 g of carbohydrate replacement fluid three hours before exercise. This does not call for candy, honey or sucrose. Those sugars before exercise resulted in reduced performance for endurance athletes. Once activity begins, minimum level of carbohydrate intake required to improve performance is 40 g per hour. One measure of carbohydrate used for fuels is respiratory exchange ratio (RER). Evidence suggests that the increase blood glucose level from taking liquid carbs before the start of exertion show respiratory ratios that increased.

The consumption of 70 to 90 g carbohydrate fluid during exertion is recommended above the 90 g threshold many individuals suffer from gastric distress. This translates to approximately 1 L of carbohydrate hydration beverage per hour. Note the rehydration component, which is stressed.

Do not use solid foods in this undertaking. Those deplete water. Hydration is your first priority. Solutions which range from 5 to 10% carbohydrates in beverages provided suitable absorption of both water and carbohydrates. Above 10% gastric emptying is inhibited. Accordingly, the recommendation is to set 5 to 10% carbohydrate rehydration beverage at the rate of 1 L per hour during exertion. For the loading regimen:

- Take a carbohydrate replacement drink containing 225 g of glucose polymers with a little glucose and fructose immediately after exertion

- Establish daily carbohydrate requirements based on body weight and exertion durations but not more than 1200 g per day and not less than 900 g per day during the course of heavy exertion.

- Eat mainly carbohydrates with low glycemic indices

- Eat carbohydrates in small meals through out the course of every day

- Used glycogen replacement drinks that are predominantly glucose polymers but also contained a small fraction of fructose

- Avoid Solids during exertion

- Habitually take 100 g of complex carbs three hours before exertion

- During the course of exertion intake 5 to 10% carbohydrate rehydration beverages at a rate of 1 L per hour

'Dieting', Diets and Diet Centres

We are continuously bombarded with anecdotal reports of individual successes [of weight loss] and not being told that most who try vigorous programmes, either drop out before completing them or regain most of if not all of the weight they have lost with time passage. Recidivism rates (weight regain to 100%+ of lost weight) on the order of 85% are to be expected even, when counseling accompanied calorie reduced approaches. Popular diet programmes disregard nutrition science: They are concerned with reducing weight rather than a correct approach - to reduce body fat. Don't strip away muscle which is the major body component that burns fat in the first place. Low Calories and/or low water diets reduce weight far too rapidly, thereby throwing the body into defensive, fat preserving reaction. The rational approach to weight reduction is only to dispose of excess body fat, while retaining muscle and body water. It has been established that diets result in 45% of the weight loss directly coming from muscle tissue. Optimisation of glycogen before actovoty is achieved through carbohydrate loading.

In a discussion of body composition for those involved in high endurance activities, many researchers have posited that there is a negative correlation between the percent of body fat presented and performance. Body-fat [above say 17%] is dead weight

For most males the optimum body fat lies between 16 and 18%. It may be slightly more in females. The measurement **methods** for body mass index for females and males are considerably different but the bottom line is the more fat you can pair off your body while preserving high levels of performance, muscle and health, the better off you will be.

Most diets rely on starvation and dehydration to 'make weight'.

Crash diets as low as 500 Cal per diem have been suggested. Another method used is to dehydrate the body dramatically to reduce 'water weight'. Both these concepts completely overlook the necessity for vitamins and minerals. Deficiencies in vitamin B6, B12, folic acid, calcium, zinc and magnesium are common with low calorie and water reduced approaches among those required to perform heavy exertion.

In 1992 the National Institute of Health reported that there is no good evidence that any popular weight loss programme has much chance of long-

Retaining muscle is essential to losing body fat that body fat Burns only minimal amounts of calories. Muscle is the first in which body fat is burned the less muscle present the Lord the basal metabolic rate, and the more difficult it is to lose fat under eating at levels of 800 and 1200 Cal does cause rapid fat loss but also occasions dramatic muscle loss. Further, it slows the med basal metabolic rate further reducing the ability to burn the fat.

Commercial diets are to be avoided since they stimulate the body to accumulate the fatty again once you stop. This under eating causes rapid fat loss as well as muscle loss and removes energy reserves that immediately takes on sorts of defensive body action. These defenses combined to decimate efforts to keep fat off. The body increases the quantity and activity of an enzyme called lipoprotein the meat pates, the main enzyme it uses to collect and store fat. In addition, it slows the basal metabolic rate further reducing the ability to burn fat.

You're asked to be where of calorie counts for foods that are contained in labeling of products on the grocery shell. To establish these levels A-bomb calorimeter is employed and the heat produced measured. Such a calorimeter is not the human body the value of 4 Cal per gram per carbohydrates and proteins and 9 Cal per gram for fats are rough approximations made up almost 100 years ago they have become entrenched and prevail as a myth in the diet industry

The value of all three major types on foods vary according to a person's biochemical individuality, affecting the digestibility, and efficiency of use of foods by each unique body. The myth of calorie intake to calorie matched weight which has long dominated American North American dieting does not work. At approximately 3600 Cal per pound; a reduction of 200 Cal per day over 18 days should result in stasis. It doesn't. Calorie counting just does not add up it has been demonstrated that fiber pills, herbal teas, artificial sweeteners, gowns, starch blockers, and grapefruit pills are of no value to weight control.

Biological Individuality and Weight Loss

As a function of biochemical individuality there is a wide range of inherited tendencies to accumulate body fat. The extrapolation that inherited proclivity demands that certain levels of fat are comfortable and healthy for individuals is dead wrong.

The habitual content of fat you carry is not predestined genetically. It reflects what you eat and what you do. Neither the number of fat cells nor their size and shape size are genetically fixed. Fatness is dependent on lifestyle. There is no reference system establishing a fixed level of fat, just a habitual level. When the individual remains at a particular level of fat for more than two years the body develops all of the adipose cells, capillaries, enzyme counts, peripheral nerves, hormone levels, and connective tissues which must support it. It comes to recognize that level of fat as self - and will defend it vigorously: that is your fat point.

Studies continue to report that it takes years to establish fat by overeating. Work slowly for permanent fat loss. Lose no more than 200 g of fat per week. This means that the individual likely will see little change in two months, but over a year the fat point edges downward by 3 to 6%. Consequently, the body is remodeling its adipose cells, hormones, enzymes capillaries and other tissues to suit the revised conditions. In this manner of resetting the fat point it does not arouse bodily defense mechanisms.

To confirm that you are losing fat and not muscles it is essential to get your body composition measured every two months. After testing dozens of systems which are proffered, it is recommended that only two: underwater weighing and infrared are reliable. This may be subject to change with technological advances. Any method will show time related 'change', if not accurate 'body fat numbers'.

The only type of food required to be removed from the diet is saturated fats. That food puts on more body fat than any other. When excess carbohydrate or proteins are eaten, the body makes complex metabolic adjustments to promote glycogen storage in muscle in increased use of protein and sugar for fuel. Hence you have to eat a big excess of these foods before they are converted to body fat when excess saturated fats are consumed virtually all the access is promptly layered into belly gets implies. Accordingly, avoid all saturated fats. These are inconveniently present in animal and dairy foods.

You are counselled to avoid commercial (book/cookbook) and weight loss centre programmes entirely.

There are of human nutrients that can assist in long-term fat wants the first of these is l-carnitine. Fats are burned for energy inside muscle cells in structures called mitochondria. However, the fats are stored in adipose cells and cannot pass through the membrane of mitochondria unless they are transported by l-carnitine. The amount of fat burned depends in large part upon this material present in the muscle. The higher the l-carnitine level, the greater the amount of body fat used for fuel. Although the body makes this, it may not make an optimum amount for heavy endurance work. This amino acid likely raises muscle carnitine levels. Accordingly maintain l-carnitine status.

A second nutrient that helps with fat reduction is the essential element chromium. While common food consumption yields less than 50 μg of chromium per day, even sedentary individuals may require 200 μg, and even moderate exercise activity demands twice that level. As a supplement between 200 and 600 μg of chromium picolinate daily is recommended.

It is important that longevists base diets on complex carbohydrates that are slowly absorbed and do not disturb insulin metabolism. For permanent fat loss reducing or eliminating sugar and eating mainly complex carbohydrates is required. High-fibre diets containing 30 to 50 g per day, create a slow even energy uptake that favors use of food for energy rather than for deposition as body fat. Insulin also remains stable. The right fibre to use is contained in the diet. Eat a high fibre diet.

It Is highly recommended that supplementation of a common diet includes chromium picolinate at 400 micrograms daily.

Two other nutrients that can help regulate insulin metabolism are the omega-3 acids found in fish oils. To achieve permanent fat loss and maintain lean mass do low intensive hydration aerobic activity daily. Do this in the morning when ever it is possible to do so. Studies have shown that exercise is raises the resting metabolic rate not only while you are doing it but for up to 18 hours afterwards. The body burns more calories per hour throughout the day but if you'd do this in the evening and then sleep the resting metabolic rate drops like a rock, and you lose the major fat loss affect. There are 14 points to permanent fat loss:

1. Lose no more than 200 to 250 g of fat per week

2. Have body-fat levels measured every two months

3. Avoid saturated fats

4. Avoid all commercial diets and 'diet centres'

5. Avoid drugs designed for weight loss (e.g. diuretics)

6. Maintain l-carnitine status

7. Maintain chromium status

8. Reduce sugars: eats complex carbohydrates

9. Eat a high fiber diet

10. Maintain omega-3 fatty acids status

11. Weight train to maintain lean mass

12. Do low intensity high duration aerobic activity daily

13. Work in the mornings above post-resting metabolic rate

14. Maintain anabolic drive

Supplementation of a Target Diet

Ageing and Supplements

During cellular metabolism, cells use oxygen to convert food into a form of energy the body can use, called ATP. Free radicals are a by-product of cellular metabolism, but it is not the only source of free radicals. Free radicals generate and are generated primarily by:

1. inflammation,
2. stress,
3. illness, and
4. ageing.

Hazardous environmental sources such as air pollution, toxic metals, alcohol, cigarette smoke, radiation, industrial chemicals, and prescribed medications expose us to more and more free radicals. Completely avoiding them is neither possible nor desirable. At low concentrations, free radicals are beneficial to the human body. Your immune system uses them to help defend itself against pathogens by stabilizing those atomic structures. When free radicals overwhelm your body, it leads to oxidative stress.

Oxidative stress is the oxidative damage that results from an imbalance between free radicals and your body's store of antioxidants. According to the free radical theory of aging, organisms age because of accumulated free radical damage to cells and DNA. The theory states that cumulative damage to cell components and connective tissue leads to wrinkles, decreased physical capability, increased susceptibility to disease, and death. While the free radical theory of aging remains controversial among some detractors, oxidative stress has been concretely demonstrated to contribute to degenerative conditions such as arthritis, heart disease, hypertension, Alzheimer's disease, Parkinson's disease, muscular dystrophy, and other disease processes.

Various studies have connected oxidative stress due to free radicals to:
- central nervous system diseases, such as Alzheimer's and other dementias
- cardiovascular disease due to clogged arteries
- autoimmune and inflammatory disorders, such as rheumatoid arthritis and cancer
- cataracts and age-related vision decline
- age-related changes in appearance, such as loss of skin elasticity, wrinkles, graying hair, hair loss, and changes in hair texture
- diabetes
- genetic degenerative diseases, such as Huntington's disease or Parkinson's

Free radicals forage through your body looking for electrons to usurp. They need pairs of electrons in order to be stable and they frantically seek molecules to achieve this. Free radicals will take (or leave) an electron, whether it's available or not, including those in fragile DNA molecules, proteins, and fats. Antioxidants defeat free radical damage to molecules by either accepting or donating an electron to make a stable atom.

Mature longevists interested in fighting free radical-related aging should avoid common sources of free radicals, such as unsuitable working conditions and ill-prepared foods. They should also eat a healthful, balanced diet supplemented with antioxidants. the mitochondrial theory of aging also asserts that free radicals damage mitochondrial DNA frequently and, over time, the damage accumulates. This regular "wear and tear" on the genetic code impedes the function of the mitochondria. When the mitochondria don't function normally, the cell doesn't receive the energy it needs and, ultimately, the operation of the cell as a whole is affected. When this happens in millions upon millions of cells, the organism itself ages and biological function begins to diminish.

Protein Supplementation

There are three basic forms of protein supplements.

- Intact proteins, such as casein the main protein in milk which are all polypeptides, many amino acids joined together.

- Hydrolysates made by putting intact proteins through an enzyme digester to break them down into individual amino acids or either dipeptide or tripeptide amino acids which are joined together

- And free-form amino acids, made by fermentation of the food in the guts of specialized bacteria

The most common drinks and meal replacement drinks available are of the first variety. They contain casein most commonly expressed in whey protein, egg protein, or soya protein in various combination. The digestive system is required to break these down into single amino acids, dipeptide's or tripeptides for absorption in the body.

The best argument for intact proteins is that the human gut evolved to digest proteins in that form. As a result, the gut initiates all sorts of essential physiologic activity in the body to respond to intact proteins. An argument can be made that they are more easily absorbed because they are predigested and would be more bio-available. The amino acid ratios of intact protein powders and hydrolysates are fixed by the amino acid of the protein employed.

The best argument for free-form amino acids mixes and the ratio of amino acids being non-fixed is that you can mix them in any ratios you prefer. If there is an ideal blend for different styles of heavy endurance work it can be made more exactly

Studies have indicated that comparing the three forms results in an edge for absorption with the second form, hydrolysates. They are absorbed faster than intact proteins. They are absorbed better than free-form amino acids because the human gut has a special transport system for dipeptide and try peptide that first from marketed supplements those that are hydrolysates rich in dipeptide and tripeptides. In this manner you will sub serve Amino acids that single amino acids cannot use. They are better retained. Other studies have shown that nitrogen retention and recovery from injury is faster with hydrolysates and with in tact proteins or equivalent free-form amino acid mixtures. They work best in the healthy guts as well as those of individuals recovering from injury.

Nitrogen retention, a measure of increase in lean tissue, was highest with whey hydrolysates. In animal studies growth was more than 220% of intact proteins and more than 600% of that on free-form amino acids. When two or more amino acids are joined together they carry information humans have separate gut systems to absorb dipeptide and tripeptides for very special reasons. The physiological response does not occur in single information-less aminos. Dipeptide and tripeptides signal the liver to produce somatedin-C, the anabolic growth factor that stimulates muscle growth.

Many manufacturers of commercial amino acid supplements concentrate their marketing on the recommended daily allowance of nine essential amino acids. This neglects the 11 non-essential amino acids that the body can make. In formation from the essential and nonessential amino acids linked together as dipeptide's signals the body to accept the protein into its store. If you leave out these latter in 11 non-essential amino acids the human body cannot retain them. Hydrolysates as predigested protein, are rich in dipeptide and tripeptides. In this manner you get an anabolic response along with your protein, and you get maximum nitrogen retention. Intact proteins and protein concentrates are 'second choices' only. They do provide the dipeptide information; but have been shown to be only half as satisfactory as hydrolysates for nitrogen retention.

Activity and Branched Chain Amino Acids

It has been established that activity causes muscles to release a large quantity of the non-essential amino acids alanine and glutamine. These amino acids are then mostly excreted from the body and lost. There is insufficient alanine and glutamine muscle to provide the quantities lost during exertion. Accordingly, much of what is released must be produced with in the muscle from other amino acids during the activity.

The three branched amino acids:

1. Leucine
2. Isoleucine
3. Valine

makeup one third of muscle protein. They are likely candidates to supply the material to make alanine. Leucine is the only one that is relatively easy to measure. There is a rapid loss of leucine during endurance activity and anaerobic activity. Studies have measured leucine oxidation in subjects indicating oxidation increases of 240% during moderate exertion. In than two hours; the leucine oxidation in one study was 90% of the total daily requirement of leucine cited in the RDA handbook. Individuals in endurance work need dramatically more.

There are three possible sources of branched chain amino acid loss during endurance activity:

1. Increase in uptake of free branched chain amino acids from the blood
2. Reduced use of branched chain amino acids in muscle protein synthesis
3. Breakdown of muscle protein

Endurance workers need to of avoid reduced muscle size and strength resulting from reduced protein synthesis - and muscle breakdown. It is therefore being essential that an adequate supply of three branched chain amino acids be present in the blood. Consuming branched chain amino acids increases blood levels - so, supplementation with these seems a sensible insurance to retaining muscle.

Quantities within Quality
Seniors Life Extension

It has been demonstrated that even sedentary persons require much more leucine than the recommended daily allowances prescribed. When leucine intakes are even 50% greater than the RDA figures, negative leucine balances are indicated. In that state muscle maintenance is not possible, and because of the principle of synergy, the status of all other amino acids is compromised. Research has concluded that the leucine requirements for healthy young sedentary persons are in the range of 20 to 40 mg per kilogram per day. For endurance workers active for more than three hours, is estimate that this requirement be at least 60 mg per kilogram per day.

When valine demand was studied with individuals presenting high endurance demands (intense exertion) a valine ingestion of 15 mg per kilogram per day was suitable.

For those in intense exertion likely requirements of 20 milligrams per kilogram of isoleucine have been reasoned from leucine demands. This is twice the current recommended daily allowance. The following table of body weight recommends these three-branch chain amino acid demands for intense activity:

- 50 kg leucine 3 g, valine 2.5 g, isoleucine 1.0 g
- 60 kg leucine 3.6 g, valine 3.0 g isoleucine 1.2 g
- 70 kg leucine at 4.2 g valine 3.5 g isoleucine 1.4 g
- 80 kg leucine at 4.8 g, valine at 4.0 g, isoleucine 1.6 g
- 90 kg leucine 5.4 g, valine at 4.5 g, isoleucine 1.8 g
- 100 kg leucine 6.0 g, valine 5.0 g, isoleucine 2.0 g

When acting on the recommended supplementation, assure that only freeform level oh amino acids are taken. Those containing the letter D indicating dextro provide a wrong direction of rotation of the chemical spiral and are ineffective. Exercise caution to obtain materials in dark glass bottles to avoid light exposure and ensure that the expiry dates are within reason before the quantity in the bottle is to be completely consumed.

Amino acids, as will all proteins, should be eaten with meals throughout the day. Endurance workers are suggested to digest no more than 30 g of protein at a single sitting. That's about six large egg whites, a chicken breast, or a can of albacore tuna – or a proteins shake take the branched chain amino acids at the same time for maximum absorption and retention. It is recommended that branched chain amino acid consumption occur one to two hours before intense exertion to spare muscle.

Vitamins

More than 40 percent of men and women in North America are hooked on multivitamins. They are the most commonly used dietary supplements. In women older than 60 years, the use of supplemental calcium has seen large increases. The use of vitamin D has increased in both men and women.

Vitamins are nutrients that every 'body' needs in small amounts to stay healthy. The amount you need depends on the vitamin. Because your body can only make limited amounts of vitamins for itself, the rest must come from a nutritious diet. Minerals are other nutrients that your body needs to function properly. Examples of commonly deficient minerals include iron, calcium and zinc. Because supplements may affect the way prescription drugs work, you should also tell your pharmacist when you begin taking them.

As you age, vitamin and mineral supplementation can keep you healthy, and retard age associated deterioration of the body. However, it is important that you use them appropriately and in conjunction with healthy diet and exercise. Exercise, far from being just a 'need' for the mature endurance workers, is in fact the impelling force behind supplementation. Consultation with a physician schooled in nutrition science and sport medicine is a requirement for the maintenance of a controlled supplementation regimen.

Vitamins are very inefficient as quick fix solutions to performance requirements. They are body and body building and maintenance prescriptions over the long haul. Vitamins are essential elements of the structure and function of the body, and take years to develop to their full capacity. Wall consuming them every day in the right amounts work regularly and consistently and the gradual changes in body makeup will be realized. All workers demand that the body continuously improve. Vitamins form one of the building materials that makes this happen. Since we know what vitamins do, the issue becomes one of whether food sources are deficient in supplying the demands required.

Vitamin A

Retinol as vitamin A has multiple functions is essential for vision skin and mucous membranes, cell growth, reproduction and immunity. It is fat-soluble, meaning that works in lipid complexes within the body it is essential for night vision. The best dietary sources of vitamin a are liver and fish oils. Best sources of beta-carotene which is a precursor of vitamin A are carrots and fresh green leafy vegetables. This alone contains three times the recommended daily allowance of vitamin a. There is widespread deficiency of vitamin A in the general population, and more so in those involved in exertion. The current recommended daily allowance provitamin a is 1000 µg of retinol equivalent. Beta-carotene is one of the few sources that is converted to vitamin A by the body. It is however a poor source because it takes six of micrograms of beta-carotene T yield 1 µg RE of vitamin A. It does have antioxidants than functions independent of its of vitamin A and therefore beta-carotene should be considered as a separate nutrient, in a reasonable amount.

A reasonable supplementation approach is 2000 µg for those in heavy endurance. This, in spite of the lack of any ergogenic affect, is recommended.

B Complex Vitamins

Vitamin B1

Vitamin B1 is a water-soluble vitamin that leaves the body daily, requiring nutrient replacement daily for optimal health. It helps to maintain normal energy metabolism. It works to burn carbohydrates. The best sources are whole grain. The thiamine content of grains may vary up to 600% depending on age, quality, storage and preparation. It's a loss from green and flowered during commercial baking can be 100%. Accordingly, the vitamin B1 your food may only be a fraction of its original content. With the high turnover of energy, endurance workers require more vitamin than the general population and are therefore likely to be deficient in this vitamin.

The recommended daily allowance for vitamin B1 at 1.5 mg per day contrasts with that recommended for workers in endurance activity of 100 mg to maintain vitamin status. Above 200 mg per day no good is indicated, it is simply secreted from the body.

Vitamin B2

Vitamin B2 as riboflavin is water-soluble. It functions to help the mitochondria of your muscles cells to produce energy. Meats poultry fish dairy are all good sources of this by food processing can damage vitamin B1 up to 8%. While the recommended daily allowance of riboflavin is 1.7 mg per day the use of 100 mg per day for endurance workers is recommended. There is no good ergogenic effect of megadoses.

Vitamin B3

Niacin as vitamin B3 is also water-soluble and is partly supplied by the diet which the body converts to function as part of two enzymes, and with a recommended daily allowance of 19 mg. For endurance workers values supplementation as niacinamide between 40 and 80 mg per day are recommended. Straight niacin may cause vascular dilation and flushing or itching. Accordingly, source as niacinamide for which tolerance is indicated. At large doses niacin blocks the use of fatty acids for fuel, so glycogen lesion occurs quickly.

Vitamin B6

Vitamin B6 as pyridine is a coenzyme which functions at all levels of protein and amino acid metabolism, as well as the manufacture of hemoglobin and all proteins. It is also essential for the enzyme glycogen phosphorylase that breaks down muscle glycogen for fuel, so the right amounts of B6 are very important for endurance workers. The best food sources are wheat germ, chicken, fish, and egg whites. You would think that these foods would make paroxetine deficiency rare. This is not the case, Requirements for vitamin B6 increase as protein requirements increase, and as the energy expenditure ramps up.

Any individual attempting to increase muscle mass who is in heavy exertion for three or more hours daily as a much higher need than the sedentary individual. While the recommended daily allowance of B6 is 2.0 mg per day, for those in higher endurance 10 mg per day is routinely accepted. Acute toxicity is low, even upwards of 200 times this level. Because of the involvement of B6 and glycogen fuel, excesses are likely to be anti-ergogenic. Megadoses of this vitamin cause a depletion in glycogen stores in muscle rapidly.

Vitamin B5

Vitamin B5 as pantheonic acid is another be complex water-soluble vitamin that has multiple roles in energy metabolism. It forms part of the co-enzyme-A and part of the carrier proteins for the enzyme fatty acid synthetase. It is necessary for making glucose and fatty acids, the main fuels of the body as well, it is essential to making steroid hormones and brain neurotransmitters. Its deficiency would point the individual in a desperate condition. It occurs widely in foods with an average intake in North America of 6 mg a day, exactly the amount deemed safe and adequate by the recommended daily allowance. That amount will not work for endurance activity. Those in intense activity use roughly 4 times the daily energy of seriously sedentary North Americans. Their need for B5 increases accordingly. Consequently, the average diet deficient for endurance workers. It is recommended that 40-80 mg of B5 be taken by those in heavy endurance work. In the form of calcium-pantothenic even at eight times this threshold (among healthy individuals), no adverse symptoms are anticipated.

Folic acid

Folate or folic acid is a B complex vitamin vital to the transport of coenzymes that control amino acid metabolism. Deficiencies inhibit growth of new cells, especially the rapidly changing muscles and blood cells of performance-geared workers. Folic acid will widely available in fresh dark vegetables, legumes and egg yolk. Poor diet has resulted in serious deficiencies among North Americans. It is the most commonly deficient of the vitamins cited here. It is fragile - and food storage and processing destroy approximately half of it found in food. The recommended daily allowance of 200 μg per day is woefully insufficient for endurance activity, especially for those intent on growing muscle to and increasing their red blood cell oxygen-carrying capacity. At this level studies of shown serious deficits of this vitamin occur. The use of minimum supplementation of 400 μg per day is recommended. Toxicity tests as high as 10000 micrograms per day were suitable.

Vitamin B12

Vitamin B12 forms part of co-enzymes essential for all cells, particularly rapid turnover cells, including red blood cells, the lining of the gastrointestinal tract and bone marrow cells. Deficiency causes pernicious anemia which disrupts nerves cells, affects mental functioning and maybe terminal. It is fortunate that severe deficiency is uncommon.

This vitamin is available only in animal foods. Vegetarians are therefore most commonly deficient. Average intake in North America is about 8 µg per day in men and 5 µg per day in women. Mega- dosing of B12 in sports has been very common. This has the best indicator of levels of B-12 is the microbiological assay, serum cobalamin. Rather than cite supplementation levels this test should indicate acceptable endurance worker levels greater than 250 pg/mL. Indicated orders of magnitude greater than the recommended daily allowance are shown to be non-toxic.

Biotin

Biotin is the last of the B complex vitamins. It forms part of the two enzymes pyruvate carboxylate and acetyl co-enzyme. As a carboxylase, biotin is essential for glucogenesis, forming new glucose and fatty acid synthesis – two major fuels for human energy. A separate biotin dependent enzyme is essential for catabolism of branched-chain amino acids. Without required biotin you can't use fat or glucose for fuel properly. You cannot break down and build up new proteins. Muscle disappears, and with deficiency you are too weak and confused to move. The best food sources for this material are liver, sardines, egg yolk and soy flour. The average diet and North Americans indicates ingestion of a less than 50 µg per day. The recommended daily allowance of the vitamin has proven labile and blood serum testing is recommended. This microbiological assay for those in heavy endurance work should show results greater than 1000 pico grams per milliliter. Oral supplementation raises blood levels quickly. Depending on measurement of serum blood content, supplementation of between 500 and 1000 micrograms per day may prove satisfactory.

Vitamin C

Vitamin C is water-soluble and accordingly quickly moves into the body and out of it. It is essential to maintain and grow white fibers of the skin, bones, and connective tissues. This is because of its action on the amino acids proline and lysine. With deficiencies skin quickly degenerates – representing the onset of scurvy. As little as 30 mg of vitamin C per day prevents this disease, but levels in excess of 1 g per day may be required to combat oxidation. Antioxidants are required for high endurance. Serum measurement above.5 mg per day is aimed for. For those in heavy work circumstances supplementation of between two and 10 g of vitamin C is recommended. We cannot avoid a reference to Dr. Linus Pauling. His research in the field of vitamin C mega-dosing was noteworthy in the 1980s and 90s. While no direct ergogenic affect of mega-dosing occurs, reduction in mean illness and injury effect appears considerable. Dr. Pauling's mental and physical health into his 90s showed that a benefit is achievable through mega-dosing of vitamin C ingestion. This may be anecdotal, but his research was not.

Vitamin D

Vitamin D is fat soluble in contrast of water solubility. It is essential for bone growth and mineral balance in the body. Exposure to sunlight synthesizes vitamin D on the skin. The recommended daily allowance of vitamin D is 10 μg daily. In healthy individuals 30 minutes per day of summer sun produces CNA only more than this. Today milk and dairy products are fortified with vitamin D extensively. Therefore, from the diet we get plenty to meet requirements. There is a risk of vitamin D toxicity at only five times the recommended daily allowance. Supplementation even for endurance work does not appear warranted if dairy products are consumed as a component of the nutritional programme, accompanied by sunlight exposure. There are no ergogenic effects on physical performance.

Vitamin E

Vitamin E is primarily a functional antioxidant. Securing quantities of vitamin E in food is rare since most is destroyed by processing. Vitamin E is a very low toxicity even at 300 times the recommended daily allowance and no side effects are demonstrated. In heavy exertion intake by supplementation of 400 to 1500 mg of output TE daily are sought. There appears to be no ergogenic effect from supplementation of these levels. Vitamin E is a basic building block of a better body.

Vitamin K

As a fat-soluble vitamin K is essential for formation of the compounds that enable blood to clot. When vitamin K is low bleeding becomes a major issue. It is therefore important of this vitamin be used in those involved in heavy exertion because continual human... Maybe cause by the exertion. Dietary sources of fresh green leafy vegetables are the best food stores providing 50 to 800 μg of vitamin K per hundred grams of food. Physical trauma such as intense muscle contraction and efforts of work increase the need for vitamin K the recommended daily allowance for vitamin K is 80 µg per diem. Because the diet can provide this with margin of comfort, supplementation above dietary demands is not directly recommended. There are concerns that supplementation of vitamin K may cause toxic side effects.

Choline

Choline is not a vitamin because the body can make it, placing it outside of the definition of vitamin it forms part of the less affluent which is an essential component of all cell membranes in every cell of the body. It is also referred to as a methyl donor in energy metabolism in the brain, choline forms part of the neurotransmitter system, intimately involved in anabolic drive and in memory. There is some evidence that megadosing of choline realizes improvement in memory of mature individuals.

Choline is widely available in foods notably from eggs, soybeans and numerous vegetables. Since the average North American daily dietary intake of 400 to 1000 mg of choline are common; supplementation of no more than 100 mg per day is reasonable. There is no evidence currently available that performance improvement or reduction in body fat is associated with choline loading.

Inositol

Myo-inositol is the form used by the body. It shapes part of the fatty components of the cell membrane. Researchers shown that is essential for normal calcium metabolism as well as insulin metabolism. It is provided to the body by food consumption and also made in the body.

Supplementation levels of 50 to 100 mg of myo-inositol for endurance workers appears both non-toxic and beneficial.

Co-enzyme Q10

Co-enzyme Q10 is essential for virtually all energy production it works by facilitating transfer of electrons in the energy cycle within the mitochondria. It is also intimately involved in maintaining immunity. It has involvements in normal heart functioning - and is a potent anti-oxidant. This fat-soluble substance, which resembles a vitamin, is present in all respiring eukaryotic cells, primarily in the mitochondria. It is a component of the electron transport chain and participates in aerobic cellular respiration, which generates energy in the form of ATP. Ninety-five percent of the human body's energy is generated this way. Considerable research, particularly in Japan, has shown efficacy with heart patients. It occurs widely in food especially in poly-unsaturated vegetable oils. The body converts it and also makes some from the amount of amino acid.

Deficiency is unlikely in sedentary individuals but in endurance workers with high energy turnover it is likely that 60 mg of coenzyme Q 10 supplementation is beneficial. No toxicity has been reported for daily consumptions in excess of 100 mg per day over a long term. In the absence of supplementation, optimal performance is unlikely.

Additional Cofactors

Bioflavonoids comprise a large family of chemicals that have numerous contributions to the human body they assist in maintaining the strength of calories are linked to vitamin C functions. They are apparently involved in the inhibition of bruising. Supplementation between 100 and 200 mg of Bible women's daily for most heavy endurance has been recommended. Cofactor PQQ is a nutrient required for normal collagen metabolism. This affects connective tissue and bone. It may be an essential nutrient and accordingly is obtained through diet. The best food source is unprocessed citrus fruit. No supplementation level for PQQ is recommended at this time

PABA is best known for its ability to prevent sunburn and skin damage by ultraviolet irradiation. Ingestion is not recommended. This product is very frequently used in the sunblock preparations. These sunscreens are highly recommended in sunlight exposure because not only is your skin affected by sunburn, but the entire immune system may be jeopardized.

A note of caution: cofactors are being hailed as today's a wonder drug. Taking 'new supplements' not mentioned in the text preceding may be a reasonable thing, but only if vitamins and cofactors are supported by concrete evidence to back them up with refereed academic research. It is more than just buyer beware: the economies can break the bank with no effect, or worse an ill-effect.

Minerals

There are five elements that make up more than 96% of the total mass of everyone's body these are:

1. Oxygen
2. Hydrogen
3. Nitrogen
4. Carbon
5. Sulfur

from dietary sources North Americans consume only 60% of that minimum amount. Maximum bone mass and bone strength occurred between the ages of 18 and 35. New regrowth and strength are however continued throughout life.

Calcium deficiency in endurance workers is tremendously important because the mineralization within bone increases dramatically in response to the stress of activity. This increased density of bone requires more calcium intake in order to make it. It is recommended that supplementation with calcium on the order of 500 to 1000 mg per day be undertaken. There is no reported toxicity for calcium intake up to 2500 mg per day. Intakes above 2500 mg per day have shown formation of kidney stones because of stress in the kidneys. Large dose intake also inhibits the absorption of iron and zinc as well; disrupting the synergy of mineral use by the body. One study found that calcium is supplementation prolonged time to exhaustion.

Magnesium

The human body contains between 20 and 30 g of magnesium, 60% in the skeleton and 40% in soft tissues. It forms a constituent of more than 300 enzymes in the body and is essential for birding glucose as fuel, transmission of genetic code, muscle contraction and many other functions which are essential. The best food sources are legumes and whole grains. However, a caveat exists in that in enriched flours and white bread have removed the germ and outer layers of the cereal grains and destroyed over 80% of the magnesium in food from grains sources.

It has been established that magnesium is one of eight nutrients required for proper metabolism of carbohydrates.

If most of the magnesium is absent because it is not added back within enriched flours, then your body has to rob tissues of magnesium in order to deal with the inadequate carbohydrates. The North American diet intake of magnesium has declined to levels of 200 to 350 mg per day, well below the recommended daily allowance of 350 mg for males and 280 mg for females. Endurance workers have more need of magnesium than sedentary individuals because of energy metabolism and muscle contraction compared to sedentary persons. They also lose abundant magnesium in perspiration. Supplementation with 400 to 1000 mg per day of magnesium is recommended there is no evidence of toxicity in healthy persons up to 6000 mg per day.

Phosphorous

There are approximately 800 g of phosphorous in a healthy body, approximately 90% of which is in bone. The balance is essential for so many other processes, from making ATP creatine phosphate (together with many other steps of the energy cycle), the metabolism of red blood cells - along with a litany of other needs. Phosphorous occurs amply in food and a lot more is added in processing in North America the best dietary sources are meats, milk, fish, and whole grains. Phosphates to have a pronounced ergogenic effect for endurance workers.

Sodium

Sodium, potassium, and chloride are three main electrolytes in the human body. They perform many essential functions without which the electrical conductance required would stop working instantly.

Sodium is the main cation [positively charged electrolyte] outside of cell structures. It is abundant in food and much is added during processing in North America frequently to levels 10 times the minimum amount recommended by the RDA handbook.

Electrolyte replacement drinks are of no value to the endurance of worker except in rare circumstances. The human body conserves its electrolytes. In endurance work the individual who sweats loses much more water than electrolyte. The needs are reflected in electrolyte overload. You need water and carbohydrates, but never sodium. Salt tablets are to be avoided totally. These pills cause salt-edemas because they force retention of water to highly unsuitable levels.

Potassium

Potassium is the main cation inside the cell structure of your body. It interfaces with sodium and chloride in a manner that conducts your impulses along with many other essential functions. Seafood has a high potassium low-sodium content. Ratios for seafood as an example are approximately 1 to 24 (sodium low to potassium high). Processing has been shown to destroy these ratios in unhealthy ways. Canned tuna is 100 parts potassium to 330 parts sodium. Commercial whole-wheat bread is 100 parts potassium two 570 parts sodium and butter is 100 parts potassium to 3600 parts sodium. For optimal performance endurance workers are counseled to stick to fresh foods wherever possible which contain enough potassium to suit body structure the average potassium intake in North America is approximately 2500 mg per day.

The recommended intake of the RDA handbook is 3500 mg per day so that even the most sedentary individuals are considerably deficient. Hemolysis and consequent losses of blood cell potassium coupled with potassium losses and sweat are consequential to endurance workers. Deficits of potassium have been demonstrated to devastate performance in marathon runners. Supplementation of potassium on the order of 100 to 500 mg per day is recommended. Potassium is not toxic up to 5000 mg per day It must be taken with food. There is no ergogenic effect from supplementation of potassium.

Chloride

Chloride is the main anion (negatively charged electrolyte) outside of so membranes. It works with two main cations, sodium and potassium to control fluid and electrolyte balance in the body the North American diet currently contains more than 600% of the recommended daily allowance for sedentary individuals. Overload, not deficiency is the problem. Chloride supplementation especially sodium chloride [table salt] is not recommended.

Iron

Iron is introduced to the body to form part of hemoglobin, the red pigment that carries oxygen in the blood stream from lungs to muscles and the brain. Iron is also a constituent of many essential enzymes. About a third of the iron in the body is stored as ferritin and hemosiderin. These materials are stored mainly in bone marrow and in the liver deficiency of this store plagues many individuals. Iron is widely available in whole grains, vegetables, meats and eggs and ends added too many processed foods that occurring in meats is most bioavailable. Iron deficiency is common throughout North America, especially so of individuals involved in endurance activity. The high incidence of deficiency is related to difficulties in absorbing it from food even the best food sources the iron is only 10% bioavailable while from vegetable sources it may only be 1% bioavailable. Calcium, fiber, and antacids all inhibit absorption further; whereas vitamin C helps you to absorb iron.

Iron supplementation on the level of 10 to 25 mg per day for endurance workers is recommended iron intakes above 100 mg per day increased risk of infection and have Betty side effects. High doses are anti-ergogenic

Zinc

Zinc forms part of numerous essential enzymes throughout the. Inadequate zinc retards muscle growth and weakens immunity. The best sources of zinc are meat, eggs and seafood. The average zinc level in the North American diet is less than 90% of the recommended daily allowance of 15 mg per day. High endurance workers need significantly more than sedentary individuals owing to their high production of red blood cells to replace cells loss by hemolysis, losses of zinc in perspiration, and the increased fatty acid metabolism involved in activity. Zinc is also involved in many interactions required for iron metabolism; and for the added testosterone required to realise muscle growth.

Because of low levels of zinc in common diets, endurance workers are doubly at risk. Supplementation of zinc at levels between 15 and 35 mg per day is recommended. Toxicity of zinc is low up to 500 mg per day. Large doses of zinc interfere dramatically with copper metabolism. They have no ergogenic effect.

Copper

Copper is required for the development of many enzymes, including those that produce noradrenalin an energizing hormone. The best sources are organ meats and seafood. Researchers shown that common North American diets provide only about 70% of the recommended daily allowance minimum adequate intake of 1.5 mg per day. Endurance workers require a greater use of copper to form noradrenalin. Supplementation is recommended at 1 mg per diem for performance.

Manganese

Manganese is required for the proper formation of bone and cartilage, for normal glucose metabolism and as a component of the endogenous anti-oxidant superoxide dismutase. It is available in food sources such as whole grains and black tea and is involved in the metabolism of carbohydrate, cholesterol and amino acids. Manganese metalloenzymes include manganese superoxide dismutase, arginase, phosphoenolpyruvate decarboxylase and glutamine synthetase. Less than 5% of dietary manganese is absorbed. In excess, it can interfere with iron absorption. Manganese deficiency may be associated with impaired growth, reproductive function and glucose tolerance as well as changes in carbohydrate and lipid metabolism. For mature workers supplementation at 5 mg per day is recommended. There is no indicated ergonomic affect to magnesium supplementation.

Chromium

Chromium is required for normal glucose metabolism, insulin metabolism, fatty acid metabolism, and muscle growth. Food storage and processing may destroy up to 90% of chromium in food sources. The best food sources for this material are whole grains and shellfish. High sugar diets deplete body tissues of chromium in order to deal with excess sugars. Chromium is rapidly depleted by exertion. In order to obtain optimal performance chromium supplementation of 200 to 500 µg per day of chromium picolinate is recommended. Chromium is an ergogenic.

Selenium

Selenium operates in conjunction with vitamin D as an antioxidant. It forms a component of the enzyme glutathione peroxidase which destroys free radicals. Many diseases including heart disease have been shown to be related to selenium and vitamin E deficiency.

Seafood and meats are the best sources of selenium. Grains, produce and animals grown on selenium deficient soils are poor sources. The recommended supplementation level for selenium is 200 to 400 µg per day for endurance workers. Selenium can be very toxic in megadosing.

Iodine

Dietary iodine is required for manufacture of thyroid hormones. As these controls all energy in the body, it is required to be precise in the quantities required. Inadequate iodine increases the size of the thyroid in response to the insufficiency. Historically iodine deficient soils resulted in severe mental retardation issues. 'Iodized' salt was introduced in order to counteract this health issue.

As a food source seafood is the best. Iodine intake in the general population as shown to be decreasing. This will likely be the result of persons reducing their intake of table salt which is treated. The average North American intake is estimated at 200 µg per day for males and 170 µg for females. This still remains above the recommended daily allowance for iodine. Endurance workers likely require more iodine and the general population because of bosses in perspiration. Supplementation levels of 50 to 200 µg per day are suggested. Iodine is not toxic up to 2000 micrograms per day. There is no ergogenic potential for iodine.

Boron

Boron provides biochemicals called hydroxyl groups, essential for the manufacture of the active form of steroid hormones: is socially hormones involved in calcium, phosphorus, and magnesium metabolism in bone, and in muscle growth. It is also required for normal testosterone production. Supplementation is recommended at levels of 3 to 5 mg per day of boron citrate and as far date toxicity of boron is low up to 50 mg per day which may interfere with phosphorus and riboflavin metabolism.

Molybdenum

Molybdenum is a component of three essential oxidase enzymes. Whole grain and leg use of the best sources available molybdenum on endurance worker recommendations for supplementation of molybdenum lie between 40 and 100 µg per day. Molybdenum has no ergogenic potential.

Antioxidants

The importance of antioxidants centres on their influence on neutralizing free radical damage to the body. There are many types of free radicals, but when we discuss them in a health capacity, we're referring to those that contain oxygen in the molecule, known collectively as *reactive oxygen species* (ROS). Oxygen is an essential element for life, and every cell in your body requires it for cellular metabolism.

Antioxidant Stability

Antioxidants are unique in that they remain stable when they donate an electron. Antioxidants sources are often discussed in terms of their free radical scavenging abilities. The "free radical scavenging activity" of antioxidants varies from one to the next. The body naturally produces some antioxidants, like glutathione, ubiquinol, and uric acid. You likely ingest many others through diet or supplements.

Some of the strongest antioxidants come from fruits and vegetables in their unique plant-based compounds called phytochemicals. Here are eight examples:

1. Anthocyanins which is found most abundantly in berries, eggplant, red cabbage, red grapes, and other richly-colored food plants, anthocyanins are purple-colored pigments common to all plants. They're what make blueberries blue and

raspberries red. Anthocyanins provide a broad range of other health benefits.
2. Polyphenols constitute a group of several thousand phytochemicals with antioxidant properties. You often hear about the polyphenols in chocolate, but scientists are pursuing and publishing more and more research on the polyphenol called curcumin, the active curcuminoid compound in turmeric.
3. Curcuminoids are polyphenol-turmeric compounds that have been recently evaluated for a myriad of health benefits. Curcuminoids protect and promote health by activating the immune system, protecting the brain, and influencing gene expression
4. Beta-carotene is a reddish orange pigment found naturally in carrots, pumpkins, sweet potatoes, mangos, spinach, squash, tomato, cantaloupe, peaches. Inside the body, it's converted into vitamin A. It's important to note that beta-carotene itself is a powerful antioxidant.
5. Lycopene is a bright red pigment found in tomatoes, watermelons, and papayas. Like beta-carotene, lycopene is a carotenoid—a type of phytochemical with antioxidant properties. Lycopene contributes to a lower risk of prostate cancer, blood clots, and stroke.
6. Vitamin C, also called ascorbic acid, supports the immune system and good health all around. It also happens to be an antioxidant. Strong contributing dietary sources of vitamin C include red and yellow bell peppers, kiwis, broccoli, cabbage, strawberries, and citrus fruits.
7. Vitamin E is a fat-soluble vitamin known for its antioxidant properties. Sunflower and safflower oil, green veggies, nuts, and seeds are rich sources of this antioxidant.

8. Selenium is an essential mineral and antioxidant that's critical for thyroid health. Our bodies do not produce selenium, so we must get it from dietary sources or supplements. Brazil nuts, button and shiitake mushrooms, lima beans, chia seeds, and brown rice are all good food sources of selenium.

Suitable endurance work performance is the product of healthy choices and a commitment to live a healthy lifestyle every single day, work day or not. There are to be no junk food compromises on non-work days. Many common foods, especially fruits and vegetables, are rich in antioxidants and a carefully planned diet should prove a good platform. External and environmental factors, however, can expose us to large quantities of free radicals: demanding increased supplementation.

Always, consult your trusted healthcare provider before increasing supplementation or changing a dosing regimen and make sure you're on track to giving your body the nutrition it needs.

Antioxidant Supplementation

The principal goal of antioxidant supplementation is the inhibition of work stress damage to all cells of the human body. Exercise generates free radicals and causes muscle damage. In the accidents have been demonstrated to prevent damage and shorten recovery time after activity. Muscle power is demonstrated in mechanical force of muscle contraction is generated by the conversion of the chemical energy of ATP. The store of 18 been in the muscles is very limited during exercise it must be regenerated continuously. The principal manner that the body does this is by conversion of muscle stores of fat and glycogen. The conversion of fat and sugar to energy occurs through oxidation. 95% of oxygen consumption does not produce many free radicals. However, the balance of 5% of oxygen use creates super oxide free radicals, hydrogen peroxide and hydroxyl free radicals. These damage every muscle they contact. The damage may cause a major source of continuing muscle soreness and weakness for days after heavy exertion.

Sports science has indicated that athletes in training, with similar demands to endurance workers, use 10 to 20 times the oxygen of sedentary persons. The free radical potential of consumptions of that quantity of oxygen are dramatic. Oxygen consumption is not the only factor in the generation of free radicals. Long endurance activity can result in a threefold increase in muscle free radicals. Supplementation with CoQ10 has shown an increase in exercise capacity on the order of 25%. This action results from the decrease in cytochrome-C activity within muscle cells.

Hydroxy radicals continue to injury your muscles long after endurance activity has stopped. The free radicals continue a process called lipid pair off oxidation. This action effectively leads to pain and inflammation. The inflammatory chain reaction of radical free radical re-formation may last up to 20 hours. Free radicals indiscriminately kill cells, poison enzymes, manufactured toxic chemicals, destroy selling are membranes with lipid peroxidation and cause the body numerous additional problems. The body fights back against oxidation by free radicals with four main forms of antioxidants:

1. Catalase which neutralizes hydrogen peroxides
2. Super-oxide dismutase which destroys superoxide radicals

3. Glutathione peroxide which detoxifies peroxides
4. Glutathione reductase

Oral supplementation for the first two of these has been demonstrated to be totally ineffective. The one major endogenous antioxidant you can manipulate nutritionally is glutathione. After exercise muscle and liver glutathione declines, indicating continued use of this antioxidant to combat free radical attack. Glutathione is produced in the body from cysteine and other amino acids. Intake of Cysteine can increase body glutathione production. As an antioxidant baseline for endurance workers a cocktail containing 300 mg of acetyl cysteine and 200 mg of L glutathione. it is noteworthy that body glutathione declines rapidly as we age. The decline in levels is so reliable that it is sometimes used as an index of the aging process.

In addition to that combination, improvement in the body's protective store of nutrient antioxidants can be achieved through supplementation by vitamin C, vitamin E, selenium and co-enzyme Q10. Vitamin E is especially valuable. Whereas glutathione protects the surfaces of cell membranes, the inside fatty membranes where the lipid peroxidation chain reaction occurs are influenced by the action fat soluble vitamin E which breaks down the chain reaction by absorbing the free radicals to form 'stable' radicals. It has been demonstrated the mineral selenium and vitamin C potentiate the activity of vitamin E in combating free radicals efficiently.

The recommended dietary allowance (RDA) of vitamin E for sedentary adults is 15 mg/d of alpha-tocopherol. This is equivalent to 22 IU (International Units) of natural source vitamin E per day, or 33 IU from synthetic sources. That is for sedentary individuals. Vigorous activity can be expected to generate three or more times the free radicals contrasted with sedentary inactivity. Accordingly, supplementation of five to eight times the RDA is reasonable for endurance workers seeking antioxidant protection from 'injury'.

The One-A-Day 'Solution'

It would be simple if taking a 'one-a-day vitamin and mineral pill' would solve endurance worker supplementation requirements. Could two, three or more of these pills bump-up the required nutritional interests of the endurance worker to levels recommended herein. This is not the case; and doing so may be dangerous.

You might go blind trying to read the fine print active constituents on bottles containing virtually all supplements - with the naked eye. A magnifying glass is required. The following is a summary of one such sample label:

- Vitamin A 300 µg
- Vitamin C 90 mg
- Formic acid 2.25 mg
- Vitamin B1 3.2 mg
- Vitamin B2 15 mg
- Vitamin B6 5 mg
- Niacinamide 15 mg `
- Vitamin B12 20
- Vitamin D3 600 international units

- Biotin 45 µg
- Pantheonic acid (B5) 10 mg
- Vitamin K 25 µg
- Calcium 200 mg
- Iodine 150 µg
- Iron 10 mg
- Magnesium 50 mg
- Copper 1000 µg
- Manganese 5 mg
- Potassium 80 mg
- Chromium 45 µg
- Molybdenum 45 µg
- Selenium 55 µg
- Zinc 7.5 mg

The Recommendations vs the 'Pill'

Now, we can contrast the individual 'pill content' with the ***baseline minimums recommended*** in the text preceding for the mature endurance worker:

- Vitamin A 300 µg present - recommended minimum 2000 micrograms: 15% of the minimum daily requirement is proffered.

- Vitamin C 90 mg present - recommended minimum 2000 mg: 4.5% of the minimum daily requirement is proffered.

- Folic acid 2.25 mcg present - recommended 400 micrograms: 0.5% of the minimum daily requirement is proffered.
- Vitamin B1 3.2 mg present - recommended 100mg: 3.2% of the minimum daily requirement is proffered.
- Vitamin B2 15 mg present - recommended 100 mg: 15% of the minimum daily requirement is proffered.
- Vitamin B6 5 mg present - recommended 10mg: 50% of the minimum daily requirement is proffered.
- Niacinamide 15 mg present - minimum recommended 40 mg: 37.5% of the minimum daily requirement is proffered.
- Vitamin B12 20 µg present - supplementation dependent on assay
- Vitamin D3 600 international units no supplementation recommended
- Biotin 45 µg present - recommended 500 micrograms: 9% of the minimum daily requirement is proffered.
- Pantheonic acid (B5) 10 mg present - recommended minimum 40mg: 25% of the minimum daily requirement is proffered.
- Vitamin K 25 µg No supplementation recommended
- Calcium 200 mg present - recommended 500 mg: 40% of the minimum daily requirement is proffered.
- Iodine 150 µg present - recommended 500 µg: 30% of the minimum daily requirement is proffered.

- Iron 10 mg present - recommended minimum 10mg: 100% of the minimum daily requirement is proffered.

- Magnesium 50 mg present - recommended minimum 400 mg: 12.5% of the minimum daily requirement is proffered.

- Copper 1000 µg present - recommended 1000 micrograms: 100% of the minimum daily requirement is proffered.

- Manganese 5 mg present - recommended 5 mg: 100% of the minimum daily requirement is proffered.

- Potassium 80 mg present - recommended minimum 100 mg: 80% of the minimum daily requirement is proffered.

- Chromium 45 µg present - recommended minimum 200 micrograms: 22.5% of the minimum daily requirement is proffered.

- Molybdenum 45 µg present - recommended minimum 40 micrograms: 100+% of the minimum daily requirement is proffered.

- Selenium 55 µg present - recommended minimum 200 micrograms: 27.5% of the minimum daily requirement is proffered.

- Zinc 7.5 mg present - recommended minimum 15 mg: 50% of the minimum daily requirement is proffered.

Several recommended supplements are not incorporated in the 'multi-vitamin with minerals' tablet presented here. What is clear is that the range of values is generally significantly below the minimum supplementation requirements for the mature endurance worker [in the case of Vitamin C only 4.5% of the *lowest threshold of supplementation*]. To get the minimum recommended level of Vitamin C, the worker would have to take 21 multi-vitamins each day – throwing other precise needs completely into uncharted territory. Taking added multi-vitamins to upgrade their highly inadequate dosing upsets all efforts to achieve 'precision'; which is the essence of endurance labour supplementation. One of these tablets might set a jumping-off point for supplementing properly, but no more than that.

Inhibiting Ageing Degradation

Research has shown that dietary calorie budgeting and introduction of antioxidants extend lifespan in various ageing models. On the one hand, oxygen is essential to all aerobic organisms because it is a final electron acceptor in mitochondria. Oxygen has been observed as harmful because it can continuously generate reactive oxygen species, which are believed to be the factors causing ageing of any biologic organism. To remove these reactive oxygen species in cells, aerobic organisms possess an antioxidant defense system which consists of a series of enzymes identified above. In addition, dietary antioxidants including ascorbic acid, vitamin A, vitamin C, α-tocopherol, and plant flavonoids are also able to scavenge reactive oxygen species in cells and therefore theoretically can extend the lifespan of organisms. Varied dietary antioxidants including:

- tea catechins,
- theaflavins,

- apple polyphenols,
- black rice anthocyanins, and
- blueberry polyphenols

have been shown to be capable of extending the lifespan of test species.

Early Stochastic Theories of Ageing

The Stochastic Theories of Ageing proposes that aging is the result of inevitable small random changes that accumulate with time and the failure of repairing stochastic damages in cells. This concept is an underly9ing principle of wear and tear theory, initially proposed by August Weismann, who believed that the ageing was due to constantly exposed to wounds, infections, and injuries and also from time to time, consuming excessive fat, sugar, and receiving undue UV lights or outsourced stresses. The accumulated damages would cause minor damages to cells and tissues, contributing to the age-related decline of organ functional efficiency. It has been revealed that animals that are raised in protected environment and do not suffer from those minor exogenous insults, still age. Later on, the theory is modified by incorporating the failure of repair hypothesis. For example, somatic mutation postulates that aging is due to alterations of chromosome number or formations of lesions in existing chromosomes, caused by accumulation of stochastic genetic mutations. Hart and Setlow add weight to development of the theory of DNA damage and repair. It is claimed that DNA damage contributes to ageing process because there is a positive correlation between DNA repair capacity and lifespan. However, nowadays STA is no longer regarded to be the sole explanation of ageing processes with a promising modified successor, free radical theory has been becoming the most widely accepted ageing mechanism hypotheses.

Energy Restriction Theory of Ageing

Energy Restriction reduces moderately nutrient availability without malnutrition. It has been shown to extend the lifespan of diverse organisms. The mechanisms of the lifespan-prolonging activity of ER in *Drosophila* were widely investigated at molecular levels. Up to date, the most recognized mechanisms for it are related to its effect on:

- metabolic rate,
- nutrient sensing insulin pathway,
- TOR pathway,
- apoptotic pathway,
- sirtuin pathway, and
- olfactory and gustatory system.

Energy Restriction has also been proposed to be associated with lesser damage of cellular macromolecules such as DNA, proteins, and lipids.

Gene expression of SOD1, SOD2, CAT, Rpn11, and Mth were studied in test organisms fed one of the three diets, namely, energy restriction diet (ER, 0.39 kcal/mL diet), standard energy diet (SE, 0.78 kcal/mL diet), and high energy diet (HE, 2.35 kcal/mL diet). Results showed that ER increased the mean lifespan by 16% compared with the control. It was demonstrated that ER group had a greater activity and gene expression of SOD1 and SOD2 than other two groups of flies. The elevated expression of Rpn11 induced by ER was observed at some time points, suggesting that the interaction of ER with Rpn11 may also mediate the lifespan-prolonging activity of ER. However, ER had no effect on the gene expression of CAT and Mth.

The Free Radical Theory of Ageing

A Free Radical Theory of Ageing was first proposed by Harman - stating that ageing is due to accumulation of oxidative damages to tissues and organs caused by free radicals. It is now considered a theorem which provides testable biological mechanism for ageing process. Reiterating, free radicals are any substances with unpaired electrons and readily react with healthy molecules in a destructive way. They can be produced in large quantities in cells by different mechanisms, such as exposure to oxygen, radiation, or environmental toxins, for example, pesticide and herbicide. The three major stages of free radical reactions are:

1. initiation,
2. propagation, and
3. termination.

No matter how it is initiated, once formed, the free radicals can propagate indefinitely in the presence of oxygen until those radicals reach a high concentration to react with each other and produce a nonradical. In general terms, any highly reactive molecules containing oxygen can be classified into this category. Reactive oxygen species are unavoidable products during normal intracellular metabolism. They actually play essential roles in cell differentiation, proliferation, and host defense response. However, their negative connotation is definitely overwhelming. Various cell components are believed to be damaged by oxygen-derived free radicals, of which three essential damages are notable:

1. lipid peroxidation, wherein reactive oxygen species can cause lipid oxidation within cells. Polyunsaturated fatty acids, the main component of

cell membranes, are vulnerable to free radical attack because they contain such multiple double bonds, which possess extremely reactive hydrogen atoms. As a result, the structure is susceptible to be attacked by free radicals, especially hydroxyl radicals, which will lead to the destruction of cell membrane permeability, and eventually the cellular dysfunction. reactive oxygen species can also damage the DNA

2. DNA damage, wherein reactives damage primarily from strand break, cross-linking, base hydroxylation, and base excision. The induction of those DNA damages will result in mutagenesis and consequently transformation, especially if combined with a deficient apoptotic pathway.

3. protein oxidation, wherein reactive oxygen species lead to the oxidation of proteins in vivo. The proteins in cells are also believed to be the main targets of free radicals. Aromatic amino acids, cysteine, and disulphide bonds are susceptible to the attack of free radicals, which will lead to protein denaturation and enzyme inactivation Furthermore, the reactive protein derivatives generated might act as intermediates to induce propagation of oxidative damages to other cell components.

Two main antioxidant systems; enzymatic antioxidants and nonenzymatic ones, act systematically to scavenge free radicals. The enzymatic antioxidant system consists of superoxide dismutase (SOD), catalase (CAT), glutathione peroxidase (GPx), and glutathione reductase (GR). This system is the main defense system against free radicals in vivo. There are two major types of SOD:

- CuZnSOD (SOD1), which mainly exist in cytoplasm, with copper and zinc being present in the active site.

- MnSOD (SOD2), located in mitochondrial matrix, with manganese being present in the active site.

These can catalyze the reaction to decompose superoxide anion radicals into H_2O_2, which will then be converted to water and oxygen by CAT or GPx. CAT is one of the most efficient redox enzymes, with iron being present in its active site, mainly found in peroxisome [10]. It can catalyze the conversion of H_2O_2 into water and oxygen. Otherwise, H_2O_2 would be converted to hydroxyl radical, one of the most active and harmful radicals to living cells. GPx is a selenium-containing enzyme, protecting cells and tissues from oxidative damage by removing H_2O_2 with the oxidization of glutathione. On the other hand, GR can convert the oxidized glutathione to its reduced form. However, the contribution of GPx in test organisms is relatively low.

Nutraceutical Life Enhancement

The term "nutraceutical" is actually a combined form of "nutrition" and "pharmaceutical." The generally accepted definition is "a food or part of a food which provides health benefits, including the prevention and/or treatment of a disease." Most nutraceuticals are dietary supplements. Studies both in vitro and in vivo reveal that consumption of nutraceuticals, especially the ones with high antioxidant capacity, has an inverse relationship with cardiovascular diseases, various cancers, and diabetes. Their contribution to 'anti-ageing activity' is yet to be quantified. On the basis of the widely accepted Free Radical Theory of Ageing - it is postulated that any substance with a great antioxidant capacity can be a potential candidate for delaying ageing. Supplements form a cornerstone of life prolongation if the theorem of Free Radical Ageing is adopted. Energy Restriction (Calorie budgeting) coupled with supplementation may extend a quality life by years - and is frankly in the best interest of all mature endurance workers.

Free Radicals and Ageing

The free radical theory of ageing is relatively recent, but numerous studies support it. Studies on test species showed *significant* increases in free radicals as they aged. These changes matched up with age-related declines in health.

There are many types of free radicals, but when we discuss them in a health capacity, we're referring to those that contain oxygen in the molecule, known collectively as *reactive oxygen species* (ROS). Oxygen is an essential element for life, and every cell in your body requires it for cellular metabolism. During cellular metabolism, cells use oxygen to convert food into a form of energy the body can use, called ATP. Free radicals are a by-product of cellular metabolism, but it is not the only source of free radicals. Free radicals generate and are generated by inflammation, stress, illness, and aging. Hazardous environmental sources such as air pollution, toxic metals, alcohol, cigarette smoke, radiation, industrial chemicals, and medications amplify the number of free radicals in the body. Completely avoiding them is neither possible nor desirable. At low concentrations, free radicals are beneficial to the human body. Your immune system uses them to help defend itself against pathogens by stabilizing those atomic structures. When free radicals overwhelm your body, it leads to oxidative stress.

Oxidative Stress

Oxidative stress is the oxidation damage that results from an imbalance between free radicals and your body's store of antioxidants. According to the free radical theory of ageing, organisms age because of accumulated free radical damage to cells and DNA. The theory states that cumulative damage to cell components and connective tissue leads to wrinkles, decreased physical capability, increased susceptibility to disease, and death. While the free radical theory of ageing remains controversial among some detractors, oxidative stress has been concretely demonstrated to contribute to degenerative conditions. Various studies have connected oxidative stress from free radicals to:

- central nervous system diseases, such as Alzheimer's and other dementias
- cardiovascular disease due to clogged arteries
- autoimmune and inflammatory disorders, such as rheumatoid arthritis and cancer
- cataracts and age-related vision decline
- age-related changes in appearance, such as loss of skin elasticity, wrinkles, graying hair, hair loss, and changes in hair texture
- diabetes
- genetic degenerative diseases, such as Huntington's disease or Parkinson's

Free radicals forage through your body looking for electrons to usurp. They need pairs of electrons in order to be stable and they frantically seek molecules to achieve this. Free radicals will take (or leave) an electron, whether it's available or not, including those in fragile DNA molecules, proteins, and fats. Antioxidants defeat free radical damage to molecules by either accepting or donating an electron to make a stable atom.

Mature workers interested in fighting free radical-related ageing should avoid common sources of free radicals, such as unsuitable working conditions and ill-prepared foods. They should also eat a healthful, balanced diet supplemented with antioxidants. the mitochondrial theory of ageing also asserts that free radicals damage mitochondrial DNA frequently and, over time, the damage accumulates. This regular "wear and tear" on the genetic code impedes the function of the mitochondria. When the mitochondria don't function normally, the cell doesn't receive the energy it needs and, ultimately, the operation of the cell as a whole is affected. When this happens in millions upon millions of cells, the organism itself ages and biological function begins to diminish.

Role of Antioxidants in Life Prolongation

Antioxidants are unique in that they remain stable when they donate an electron. Antioxidants sources are often discussed in terms of their free radical scavenging abilities. The "free radical scavenging activity" of antioxidants varies from one to the next. The body naturally produces some antioxidants, like glutathione, ubiquinol, and uric acid. You likely ingest many others through diet or supplements.

Some of the strongest antioxidants come from fruits and vegetables in their unique plant-based compounds called phytochemicals. Here are eight examples:

9. Anthocyanins which is found most abundantly in berries, eggplant, red cabbage, red grapes, and

other richly-colored food plants, anthocyanins are purple-colored pigments common to all plants. They're what make blueberries blue and raspberries red. Anthocyanins provide a broad range of other health benefits.
10. Polyphenols constitute a group of several thousand phytochemicals with antioxidant properties. You often hear about the polyphenols in chocolate, but scientists are pursuing and publishing more and more research on the polyphenol called curcumin, the active curcuminoid compound in turmeric.
11. Curcuminoids are polyphenol-turmeric compounds that have been recently evaluated for a myriad of health benefits. Curcuminoids protect and promote health by activating the immune system, protecting the brain, and influencing gene expression
12. Beta-carotene is a reddish orange pigment found naturally in carrots, pumpkins, sweet potatoes, mangos, spinach, squash, tomato, cantaloupe, peaches. Inside the body, it's converted into vitamin A. It's important to note that beta-carotene itself is a powerful antioxidant.
13. Lycopene is a bright red pigment found in tomatoes, watermelons, and papayas. Like beta-carotene, lycopene is a carotenoid—a type of phytochemical with antioxidant properties. Lycopene contributes to a lower risk of prostate cancer, blood clots, and stroke.
14. Vitamin C, also called ascorbic acid, supports the immune system and good health all around. It also happens to be an antioxidant. Strong contributing dietary sources of vitamin C include red and yellow bell peppers, kiwis, broccoli, cabbage, strawberries, and citrus fruits.
15. Vitamin E is a fat-soluble vitamin known for its antioxidant properties. Sunflower and safflower oil,

green veggies, nuts, and seeds are rich sources of this antioxidant.
16. Selenium is an essential mineral and antioxidant that's critical for thyroid health. Our bodies do not produce selenium, so we must get it from dietary sources or supplements. Brazil nuts, button and shiitake mushrooms, lima beans, chia seeds, and brown rice are all good food sources of selenium.

Life enhancement is the product of healthy choices and a commitment to live a healthy lifestyle every single day, week-end or not. There are to be no junk food compromises or 'holidays'. Many common foods, especially fruits and vegetables, are rich in antioxidants and a carefully planned diet should prove a good platform. External and environmental factors, however, can expose us to large quantities of free radicals: demanding increased supplementation.

Always, consult your trusted healthcare provider before increasing supplementation or changing a dosing regimen and make sure you're on track to giving your body the nutrition it needs.

Rationalising a Programme of Exercise for Health Outcome

Exercise Physiologists and researchers have long been interested in:

- how much time and 'in group' exercise is optimal
- what types (modes) of exercise are optimal
- can exercise slow or reverse ageing processes

These questions have only recently been scrutinized scientifically. It is recognised that no one amount or type of exercise is likely to be best for every health benefit.

Early research has shown resistance training to improve glucose tolerance and glycosylated hemoglobin, as well as strength and lean body mass. Its influence on other metabolic variables was less clear. Of considerable interest to both the longevist community and the scientific community is the control of weight gain and the extent of weight loss and change in body composition induced by exercise training. One 2012 comprehensive research study [Willis et. al.] investigated the relative benefits of resistance training when compared with aerobic training and the combination of the two on body composition measures, particularly total body mass and fat mass. That study directly compared changes in body composition induced by comparable amounts of time spent doing resistance and aerobic training, or both in combination, in nondiabetic, previously inactive overweight or obese adults.

Although resistance training and aerobic training are vastly different in terms of the nature of the training stimulus, specifically;

1. intermittent vs. continuous contractions,
2. time skeletal muscle is under load,

3. metabolic pathways utilized,
4. other factors,

The basis for comparison was that the prescriptions utilised were consistent with national recommendations for the 'general population'. The main findings of the 2012 study reached the following four conclusions:

1. A substantial amount of resistance training alone did not reduce body mass or fat mass;
2. recommended amounts of aerobic training were significantly better than resistance training for reducing measures of body fat and body mass; and
3. the combination of aerobic and resistance training did not provide an additive effect for reducing fat mass or body mass compared with aerobic training alone.
4. training modes in combination neither acted in synergy nor interfered but rather seemed to act in a linear fashion when body composition measures were the outcome variables.

Resistance Training

The resistance training exercise prescription used in the study was the upper limit of the amount recommended by the American College of Sports Medicine in terms of both sessions per week and number of sets per session resistance training induced significant gains in lean body mass and strength. The lack of body mass loss observed with resistance training in this study supports the findings of others and is driven by an increase in lean body mass. However, there are conflicting reports in the literature on whether or not resistance training induces fat mass loss: some randomized controlled trials find that resistance training significantly reduces fat mass while others either report a statistically insignificant trend (or no change in fat mass). The 2012 study supports the latter observation. However, it should be emphasized that resistance training significantly ($P < 0.05$) improved lean body mass as confirmed by both BOD POD and thigh muscle area measurements.

Recommendations from the American College of Sports Medicine (2009) provide a figure that proposes three potential mechanisms by which resistance training might lead to fat mass loss. Although the authors state that the literature examining the effect of resistance training on fat mass is inconclusive and that resistance training is not effective for weight loss, *resistance training is still endorsed by those authors as an effective means for obesity treatment*. Similarly, other consensus documents and study reports include tables showing that resistance training results in decreases in fat percentage, with the suggestion that this decrease in fat percent indicates a decrease in fat mass. The problem with reporting changes in fat percent, instead of absolute fat mass, is demonstrated by the resistance training group in the 2012 study, for whom fat percent did significantly decrease without any change in absolute fat mass. In other words, the changes in percent body fat were driven solely by the increase in lean body mass induced with resistance training. That study failed to observe significant total body or fat mass loss even with a very substantial resistance training programme of 8-month duration.

Perhaps the most commonly cited reason for the reduction of fat mass and body weight by resistance training is that resting metabolic rate (RMR) theoretically increases as lean body mass increases, resulting in a steady state increase in total energy expenditure and a negative shift in energy balance. Although it did not directly measure RMR it was observed that resistance training increased lean body mass without a significant change in fat mass or body weight, irrespective of any change in RMR that might have occurred. Given these observations, along with those from other studies it may be time to seriously reconsider the conventional wisdom that resistance training alone can induce changes in body mass or fat mass due to an increase in metabolism in overweight or obese sedentary adults.

Comparing Aerobic and Resistance Training

It is important for the longevist to understand whether aerobic or resistance training is superior in inducing changes in overall body composition. Comparisons between aerobic training and resistance training groups in the 2012 study suggest that aerobic training decreases both body weight and fat mass significantly more than does resistance training. While the two modes of exercise produced statistically similar changes in body fat percentage, these changes were driven by different mechanisms, where resistance training increased lean body mass and aerobic training decreased fat mass. These data are supported by other findings from that enquiry indicating that aerobic training significantly reduced visceral adipose tissue more than resistance training and trended toward the same result in liver fat change. Additionally, the 2012 study suggests that aerobic training trended toward significantly improving metabolic syndrome score better than resistance training. Furthermore, another meta-analysis of aerobic vs. resistance training effects on visceral fat concluded that there is a trend toward a greater reduction in visceral fat with aerobic training when compared to resistance training. These data, taken together and combined with the knowledge that the resistance training programme in was equivalent to the top end of those suggested in recent the exercise duration in the combined group was approximately twice that of the aerobic training [alone] group.

Waist circumference.

There is increasing evidence that central obesity is more strongly correlated with cardiovascular disease than measures of general obesity, such as BMI and body mass. It is important therefore to note that the combined aerobic training+resistance training exercise group decreased minimal waist circumference significantly more than did resistance training. Perhaps the significant increase in exercise duration for the combined group explains this finding. However, the aerobic training group toward significantly decreased waist circumference by a greater increment than did resistance training and as previously stated, the time commitment was similar between these groups.

The data of the 2012 study points to the following four conclusions:

1. Although it was more effective for lean body mass gains, resistance training did not significantly reduce either fat mass or total body mass.
2. Aerobic training was more effective than resistance training for the reduction of fat and body mass in previously sedentary, nondiabetic, overweight or obese adults.
3. While requiring double the time commitment, a programme of combined aerobic training and resistance training did not result in a greater loss of fat mass or body mass over aerobic training on its own.

4. If increasing muscle mass and strength is the goal, a programme including resistance training is required. However, balancing time commitments against health benefits accrued, it appears that aerobic training alone is the optimal mode of exercise for reducing fat mass and total body mass.

Brain Size and Functional Benefits of Aerobic Exercise

The hippocampus shrinks in late adulthood, leading to impaired memory and increased risk for dementia. Hippocampal volume shrinks 1–2% annually in older adults without dementia, and this loss of volume increases the risk for developing cognitive impairment. Hippocampal and medial temporal lobe volumes are larger in higher-fit adults, and physical activity training increases hippocampal perfusion, but the extent to which aerobic exercise training can modify hippocampal volume in late adulthood remains unquantified. Ericson, Voss et al., in a 2011 demonstrated that in a randomized controlled trial with 120 older adults, that aerobic exercise training increases the size of the anterior hippocampus, leading to improvements in spatial memory. Exercise training increased hippocampal volume by 2%, effectively *reversing* age-related loss in volume by 1 to 2 y. We also demonstrate that increased hippocampal volume is associated with greater serum levels of BDNF, a mediator of neurogenesis in the dentate gyrus. Hippocampal volume declined in the control group, but higher preintervention fitness partially attenuated the decline, suggesting that fitness protects against volume loss.

These theoretically important findings indicate that aerobic exercise training is effective at reversing hippocampal volume loss in late adulthood, which is accompanied by improved memory function. Study results showed consistency with the shrinkage pattern, such that the stretching control group demonstrated a 1.4% decline in volume over the 1-y interval. With escalating health care costs and an increased proportion of people aged >65 y, it is imperative that low-cost, accessible preventions and treatments for brain tissue loss are discovered. In this randomized controlled study of exercise training, Ericsson et al. demonstrate that loss of hippocampal volume in late adulthood is not inevitable and can be reversed with moderate-intensity exercise. A 1-y aerobic exercise intervention was effective at increasing hippocampal volume by 2% and offsetting the deterioration associated with aging. Because hippocampal volume shrinks 1–2% annually, a 2% increase in hippocampal volume is equivalent to 'restoring' between 1 and 2 y worth of volume to the hippocampus for this age group.

Aerobic exercise increased anterior hippocampal volume but had little effect on the posterior hippocampus. Neurons in the anterior hippocampus are selectively associated with spatial memory acquisition and show exacerbated age-related atrophy compared with the posterior hippocampus. Thus, aerobic exercise might elicit the greatest changes in regions that show the most precipitous decline in late adulthood, such as the anterior hippocampus and prefrontal cortex. Overall, these data suggest that the anterior hippocampus remains amenable to augmentation.

Strategies to fight hippocampal loss and protect against the development of memory impairment has become an important topic in recent years from both scientific and public health perspectives. Physical activity, such as aerobic exercise, has emerged as a promising low-cost treatment to improve neurocognitive function that is accessible to most adults and is not plagued by intolerable side effects frequently found with pharmaceutical interventions.

Aerobic exercise training increases gray and white matter volume in the prefrontal cortex of older adults and increases the functioning of key nodes in the executive control network Greater amounts of physical activity are associated with sparing of prefrontal and temporal brain regions over a 9-year period, which reduces the risk for cognitive impairment. Further, hippocampal and medial temporal lobe volumes are larger in higher-fit older adults, and larger hippocampal volumes mediate improvements in spatial memory. Exercise training increases cerebral blood volume and perfusion of the hippocampus, but the extent to which exercise can modify the size of the hippocampus in late adulthood remains unknown.

Study results demonstrate that the size of the hippocampus is modifiable in late adulthood and that moderate-intensity aerobic exercise is effective at reversing volume loss. Increased volume with exercise occurred in a selective fashion, influencing the anterior hippocampus but not the posterior hippocampus or the thalamus or caudate nucleus.

Changes in Fitness Are Associated with Increased Hippocampal Volume.

The intervention was effective at increasing aerobic fitness levels. The aerobic exercise group showed a 7.78% improvement in maximal oxygen consumption (VO_2 max) after the intervention, whereas a 'stretching control group' showed a 1.11% improvement in VO_2 max. Improvements in fitness levels were associated with the magnitude of the change in hippocampal volume.

increased hippocampal volume was directly related to improvements in memory performance. The correlation between improvement in memory and hippocampal volume reached significance for left) and right hemispheres. This indicates that increases in hippocampal volume after 1 year of exercise augments memory function in late adulthood.

Introducing an Aerobic Programme for Seniors

Regular cardio exercise is important for any age group, but older adults probably have the most to gain from starting (or continuing) an exercise program. Aerobic exercise has been shown to:

- strengthen heart and lungs,
- Yields you more energy,
- sharpens cognition, helps manage weight,
- can reduce symptoms of anxiety and depression, and
- may extend life expectancy.

The question often is, how much 'work' should you do, and what's the best way to get started? The ACSM/AHA Physical Activity Recommendations for Older Adults suggest three different options:

- Moderate intensity cardio for 30 minutes, 5 days a week, or
- Vigorous cardio for 20 minutes, 3 days a week, or
- A mix of moderate and vigorous cardio, 3-5 days a week

Setting Up Your Cardio Workouts

The recommendations sound simple but making them a reality can be confusing. Use these steps to set up your cardio workout:

1. **Choose an Activity** - Pick any activity where you can work at a moderate or vigorous intensity level (or about

65% to 80% of your maximum heart rate). Choose something you enjoy, that's accessible, and that fits your needs. For example, if you have joint pain or problems, you might prefer a low to no-impact exercise like swimming or biking. There are nine common options, which can be done indoors or outdoors:

1. Walking
2. Running
3. Stepping (machine)
4. Cycling
5. Rowing (machine)
6. Elliptical (machine)
7. Swimming
8. Aerobics and Aerobic Dance
9. Home exercise videos

2. **Choose How Long to Exercise** - While the ACSM recommends 20-30 minutes, you may need to work up to that if you haven't exercised before. It takes time to build endurance in your heart and muscles, so start with what you can handle and add a few minutes to each workout to work your way up gradually. For example, a beginner might start with 10-15 minutes of walking or cycling and build from there.

3. **Choose Your Intensity** - The guidelines suggest moderate intensity, which is around Level 5-6 on this perceived exertion scale. Start with a comfortable pace to get a feel for the exercise. Once you feel comfortable, you can push a little harder. Basically, you want to work at a level

where you can talk, but only in short sentences. A great way to work on endurance without having to work hard the entire workout is with interval training. Try walking fast for 1 minute and then slowing down a bit for 1-2 minutes, alternating that for 20 or so minutes.

4. **Choose How Often You Exercise** - If you're a beginner or not sure what you can handle, start with three days a week with rest days in between. You can add more days once you feel ready for more frequent exercise.

For Seniors, guidelines suggest working up to one of the following options:

- Moderate Intensity of 150 minutes per week (5 days of 30 minutes work)
- Vigorous Intensity 75 minutes per week (3 days of 25 minutes work)

Selected Readings

- Gordijn B. *Medical utopias: ethical reflections about emerging medical technologies.* Leuven: Peeters, 2006
- Harris J. *Immortal ethics.* Ann N Y Acad Sci 20041019527–534.
- Glannon W. *Extending the human life span.* J Med Philos 200227339–354.
- Harris J, Holm S. *Extending human life span and the precautionary paradox.* J Med Philos 200227355–368.
- Davis J K. *Collective suttee: is it unjust to develop life extension if it will not be possible to provide it to everyone?* Ann N Y Acad Sci 20041019535–541
- Juengst E T, Binstock R H, Mehlman M J. et al *Aging: Antiaging research and the need for public dialogue.* Science 20032991323
- Juengst E T, Binstock R H, Mehlman M. et al *Biogerontology, "anti-aging medicine," and the challenges of human enhancement.* Hastings Cent Rep 20033321–30.
- Dwyer J. *Global health and justice.* Bioethics 200519460–475.
- Benatar S. *Bioethics: power and injustice*: IAB presidential address. Bioethics 200317387–398.
- Dwyer J. *Teaching global bioethics.* Bioethics 200317432–446
- Farmer P, Gastineau Campos N. *Rethinking medical ethics: a view from below.* Developing World Bioeth 2004417–41.
- Davis J K. *The prolongevists speak up: the life-extension ethics session at the 10th Annual Congress of the International Association of*

- Biomedical Gerontology. Am J Bioeth 20044W6–W8.
- Lucke J, Hall W. *Who wants to live forever?* EMBO Rep 2005698–102.
- McCay CM, Crowel MF, Maynard LA. *The effect of retarded growth upon the length of the life span and upon the ultimate body size.* J Nutr 1935;10; 63–79.
- Barrows CH, Kokkonen GC. *Dietary restriction and life extension, biological mechanisms .* In: Moment GB, ed. Nutritional approaches to aging research. Boca Raton, Fl CRC Press Inc, 1982: 219–43
- Weindruch R, Walford RL. *The retardation of aging and disease by dietary restriction.* Springfield, IL: Charles C Thomas Publisher, 1988
- Roth GS, Lane MA, Ingram DK, et al. *Biomarkers of caloric restriction may predict longevity in humans* Science 2002; 297:811.
- Kemnitz JW, Weindruch R, Roecker EB, Crawford K, Kaufman PL, Ershler WB. *Dietary restriction of adult male rhesus monkeys: design, methodology, and preliminary findings from the first year of study* J Gerontol1993; 48 B17–26
- Mazat L, Lafont S, Berr C, et al. *Prospective measurements of dehydroepiandrosterone sulfate in a cohort of elderly subjects: relationship to gender, subjective health, smoking habits, and 10-year mortality.* Proc Natl Acad Sci U S A 2001;98
- Committee on a National Research Agenda on Aging. Extending life, enhancing life: a national research agenda on aging. Washington, DC: National Academy Press,1991
- Martorell R *Interrelationships between diet, infectious disease, and nutritional status* In: Greene LS, Johnston FE, eds. Social and biological

predictors of nutritional status, physical growth, and neurological development. New York: Academic Press, 1980: 81–106
- Ulijaszek SJ. *Nutritional status and susceptibility to infectious disease* In: Waterlow JC, ed. Diet and disease. New York: Cambridge University Press, 1990: 137–54
- Villeneuve PJ, Morrison HI, Craig CL, Schaubel DE. *Physical activity, physical fitness, and risk of dying.* Epidemiology 1998;9: 626–3
- Sohal RS, Weindruch R. *Oxidative stress, caloric restriction, and aging.* Science1996; 273: 59–63
- Meites J. *Evidence that underfeeding acts via the neuroendocrine system to influence aging processes.* Prog Clin Biol Res 1989; 287: 169–80

- McCarter R, Masoro EJ, Yu BP.*Does food restriction retard aging by reducing the metabolic rate?* Am J Physiol 1985; 248:
- E488–90
- Lynn WS, Wallwork JC. *Does food restriction retard aging by reducing metabolic rate?* J Nutr 1992; 122: 1917–8
- Poehlman ET, Melby CL, Badylak SF. *Relation of age and physical exercise status on metabolic rate in younger and older healthy men.* J Gerontol 1991;46:B54–8
- Fricker J, Rozen R, Melchior JC Apfelbaum M. *Energy-metabolism adaptation in obese adults on a very-low-calorie diet.* Am J Clin Nutr 1991;53:826–30
- Leibel RL, Rosenbaum M, Hirsch J. *Changes in energy expenditure resulting from altered body weight.* N Engl J Med1995;332:621–8

- Sohal RS, AllenRG. *Relationship between metabolic rate, free radicals, differentiation and aging: a unified theory.* Basic Life Sci1985;35:75–104
- Orr WC, Sohal RS. *Extension of life-span by overexpression of superoxide dismutase and catalase in Drosophila melanogaster.* Science1994;263:1128–30
- Melov S, Ravenscroft J, Malik S, et al. *Extension of life-span with superoxide dismutase/catalase mimetics.* Science 2000;289:1567–9
- Lee DW, Yu BP. *Modulation of free radicals and superoxide dismutases by age and dietary restriction.* Aging (Milano) 1990; 2:357–62
- Bohr VA, Dianov GL. *Oxidative DNA damage processing in nuclear and mitochondrial DNA.* Biochimie 1999;81:155–60
- Loft S, Astrup A, Buemann B, Poulsen HE. *Oxidative DNA damage correlates with oxygen consumption in humans.* FASEB J 1994;8: 534–7
- Lev-Ran A. *Mitogenic factors accelerate later-age diseases: insulin as a paradigm.* Mech Ageing Dev 1998 102:95–113
- Jennings B, Callahan D, Wolf S M. *The professions: public interest and common good.* Hastings Cent Rep 1987173–10.
- Barazetti, Gaia (2011*), "Looking for the Fountain of Youth: Scientific, Ethical, and Social Issues in the Extension of Human Lifespan"*, in Julian Savulescu, Ruud ter Meulen, and Guy Kahane (eds.), Enhancing Human Capacities (Oxford: Wiley-Blackwell).
- Barazetti, Gaia and Massimo Reichlin (2011*), "Life-extension and Personal Identity"*, in Julian Savulescu, Ruud ter

- Meulen, and Guy Kahane (eds.), *Enhancing Human Capacities* (Oxford: Wiley-Blackwell).
- Baumer, Yvonne, Beate Scholz, Svetlana Ivanov, and Burkhard Schlosshauer (2011), *"Telomerase-Based Immortalization Modifies the Angiogenic/Inflammatory Responses of Human Coronary Artery Endothelial Cells"*, Experimental Biology and Medicine, 236 (6), 692-700.
- Blackford, Russell (2009), *"Moral Pluralism Versus the Total View: Why Singer Is Wrong About Radical Life extension"*, Journal of Medical Ethics, 35 (12), 747-52.
- Harley, Jerry W. Shay, Serge Lichtsteiner, and Woodring E. Wright (1998), *"Extension of Lifespan by Introduction of Telomerase into Normal Human Cells"*, Science, 279 (5349), 349-52.
- Bostrom, Nick and Toby Ord (2006), "*The Reversal Test: Eliminating Status Quo Bias in Applied Ethics*", Ethics, 116 (4), 656-79.
- Buchanan, Allen (2011), *Beyond Humanity? The Ethics of Biomedical Enhancement* (Oxford: Oxford University Press).
- Callahan, Daniel (1994), *"Manipulating Human Life: Is There No End in It?"*, in Robert H. Blank and Andrea L. Bonnicksen (eds.), Medicine Unbound: The Human Body and the Limits of Medical Intervention (New York: Columbia University Press).
- Camerer, Colin F. and Howard Kunreuther (1989), *"Decision Processes for Low Probability Events: Policy Implications"*, Journal of Policy Analysis and Management, 8 (4), 565-92.
- de Grey, Aubrey D. N. J. (2005), *"Life-extension, Human Rights, and the Rational Refinement of

Repugnance", Journal of Medical Ethics, 31 (11), 659-63.
- Dohmen, Thomas J., Armin Falk, David Huffman, Uwe Sunde, Jürgen Schupp, and Gert G. Wagner (2005), *'Iza Discussion Paper No. 1730: Individual Risk Attitudes: New Evidence from a Large, Representative, Experimentally-Validated Survey'*, (Bonn: Institute for the Study of Labor).
- Finch, Caleb E. (2009), *"Update on Slow Aging and Negligible Senescence: A Mini-Review"*, Gerontology, 55 (3), 307-13.
- Fukuyama, Francis (2002*), Our Posthuman Future: Consequences of the Biotechnology Revolution* (New York: Picador).20
- Gems, David (2003), *"Is More Life Always Better? The New Biology of Aging and the Meaning of Life"*, The Hastings Center Report, 33 (4), 31-39.
- Glannon, Walter (2002a), *"Extending the Human Life Span"*, Journal of Medicine and Philosophy, 27 (3), 339-54.
- Green, Leonard, Astrid Fry, and Joel Myerson (1994), *"Discounting of Delayed Rewards: A Lifespan Comparison"*, Psychological Science, 5 (1), 33-36.
- Habermas, Jürgen (2003*), The Future of Human Nature* (Cambridge: Polity Press).
- Hackler, Chris (2004), *"Extending the Life Span: Mythic Desires and Modern Dangers"*, HEC Forum, 16 (3), 182-96.
- Harris, John (2002a), *"Intimations of Immortality: The Ethics and Justice of Life Extending Therapies"*, in Michael Freeman (ed.), Current Legal Problems (Oxford: Oxford University Press).

- Horrobin, Steven (2006), "Immortality, Human Nature, the Value of Life and the Value of Life-extension", Bioethics, 20 (6), 279-92.
- Jaskelioff, Mariela, Florian L. Muller, Ji-Hye Paik, Emily Thomas, Shan Jiang, Andrew C. Adams, Ergun Sahin, Maria Kost-Alimova, Alexei Protopopov, Juan Cadinanos, James W. Horner, Eleftheria Maratos-Flier, and Ronald A. DePinho (2011), "Telomerase Reactivation Reverses Tissue Degeneration in Aged Telomerase Deficient Mice", Nature, 469 (6 January 2011), 102-06.
- Kass, Leon R. (2001), "L'chaim and Its Limits: Why Not Immortality?", First Things, (May 2001), 17-24.
- Marshall, Jennifer (2006), "Life-extension Research: An Analysis of Contemporary Biological Theories", Medicine, Health Care and Philosophy, 9 (1), 87-96.21
- McKibben, Bill (2003), *Enough: Genetic Engineering and the End of Human Nature* (London: Bloomsbury).
- Overall, Christine (2003), *Aging, Death, and Human Longevity: A Philosophical Inquiry* (Berkeley: University of California Press).
- Ruan, Hongyu, Xiang Dong Tang, M. L. Chen, M. A. Joiner, Guangrong Sun, Nathan Brot, Herbert Weissbach, Stephen H. Heinemann, Linda Iverson, Chun-Fang Wu, and Toshinori Hoshi (2002), "High-Quality Life extension by the Enzyme Peptide Methionine Sulfoxide Reductase", Proceedings of the National Academy of Sciences of the United States of America, 99 (5), 2748-53.
- R. Weindruch, R.S. Sohal *Caloric intake and aging* N. Engl. J. Med., 337 (1997), pp. 986-994

- F.M. Cerqueira, A.J. Kowaltowski *Mitochondrial metabolism in aging: effect of dietary interventions* Ageing Res. Rev., 12 (2013), pp. 22-28
- W. Mair, A. Dillin *Aging and survival: the genetics of life span extension by dietary restriction* Annu. Rev. Biochem., 77 (2008), pp. 727-754
- A.M. Holehan, B.J. Merry *The experimental manipulation of aging by diet* Biol. Rev., 61 (1986), pp. 329-368
- R. Weindruch, R.L. Walford *The Retardation of Aging and Disease by Dietary Restriction* Thomas, Springfield, IL (1988)
- E.J. Masoro *Caloric Restriction: a Key to Understanding and Modulating Aging* Elsevier, Amsterdam (2002)
- B.P. Yu *Aging and oxidative stress: modulation by dietary restriction* Free Radic. Biol. Med., 21 (1996), pp. 651-668
- L. Fontana, L. Partridge, V.D. Longo *Extending healthy life span—from yeast to humans* Science, 328 (2010), pp. 321-326
- E.J. Masoro *Overview of caloric restriction and ageing* Mech. Ageing Dev., 126 (2005), pp. 913-922
- S.D. Morrison *Nutrition and longevity* Nutr. Rev., 41 (1983), pp. 133-142
- W.R. Swindell *Dietary restriction in rats and mice: a meta-analysis and review of the evidence for genotype-dependent effects on lifespan* Ageing Res. Rev., 11 (2012), pp. 254-270
- C.Y. Liao, B.A. Rikke, T.E. Johnson, V. Diaz, J.F. Nelson *Genetic variation in the murine lifespan response to dietary restriction: from life extension to life shortening* Aging Cell, 9 (2010), pp. 92-95

- Turturro, W.W. Witt, S. Lewis, B.S. Hass, R.D. Lipman, R.W. Hart *Growth curves and survival characteristics of the animals used in the Biomarkers of Aging Program* J. Gerontol. A Biol. Sci. Med. Sci., 54 (1999), pp. B492-B501
- W.G. Sheldon, T.J. Bucci, B. Blackwell, A. Turturro *Effect of ad libitum feeding and 40% feed restriction on body weight, longevity and neoplasms* in B6C3F1, C57BL/6, and B6D2F1 mice
- B.N. Blackwell, T.J. Bucci, R.W. Hart, A. Turturro *Longevity, body weight, and neoplasia in ad libitum-fed and diet-restricted C57BL6 mice fed NIH-31 open formula diet* Toxicol. Pathol., 23 (1995), pp. 570-582
- Wang, R. Weindruch, J.R. Fernandez, C.S. Coffey, P. Patel, D.B. Allison *Caloric restriction and body weight independently affect longevity in Wistar rats* Int. J. Obes. Relat. Metab. Disord., 28 (2004), pp. 357-362
- H.R. Warner, G. Fernandes, E. Wang *A unifying hypothesis to explain the retardation of aging and tumorigenesis by caloric restriction* J. Gerontol. A Biol. Sci. Med. Sci., 50 (1995), pp. B107-B109
- R. Weindruch, R.L. Walford, S. Fligiel, D. Guthrie *The retardation of aging in mice by dietary restriction: longevity, cancer, immunity and lifetime energy intake* J. Nutr., 116 (1986), pp. 641-654
- E.J. Masoro *Caloric restriction-induced life extension of rats and mice: a critique of proposed mechanisms* Biochim. Biophys. Acta, 1790 (2009), pp. 1040-1048
- F.L. Muller, M.S. Lustgarten, Y. Jang, A. Richardson, H. Van Remmen *Trends in oxidative*

aging theories Free Radic. Biol. Med., 43 (2007), pp. 477-503

- J.J. Ramsey, M.E. Harper, R. Weindruch *Restriction of energy intake, energy expenditure, and aging* Free Radic. Biol. Med., 29 (2000), pp. 946-968
- J.R. Speakman, S.E. Mitchel *Caloric restriction* Mol. Aspects Med., 32 (2011), pp. 159-221
- M.E. Walsh, Y. Shi, H. Van Remmen *The effects of dietary restriction on oxidative stress in rodents* Free Radic. Biol. Med., 66 (2014), pp. 88-99
- R.J. Mockett, T.M. Cooper, W.C. Orr, R.S. Soha *Effects of caloric restriction are species-specific* Biogerontology, 7 (2006), pp. 157-160
- S. Nakagawa, M. Lagisz, K.L. Hector, H.G. Spencer *Comparative and meta-analytic insights into life extension via dietary restriction* Aging Cell., 11 (2012), pp. 401-409
- S.J. Simpson, D. Raubenheimer *Macronutrient balance and lifespan Aging*, 1 (2009), pp. 875-880
- S.J. Simpson, D. Raubenheimer *Caloric restriction and aging revisited: the need for a geometric analysis of the nutritional bases of aging* J. Gerontol. A Biol. Sci. Med. Sci., 62 (2007), pp. 707-713
- S.M. Solon-Biet, A.C. McMahon, J.W. Ballard, K. Ruohonen, L.E. Wu, V.C. Cogger, A. Warren, X. Huang, N. Pichaud, R.G. Melvin, R. Gokarn, M. Khalil, N. Turner, G.J. Cooney, D.A. Sinclair, D. Raubenheimer, D.G. Le Couteur, S.J. Simpson *The ratio of macronutrients, not caloric intake, dictates cardiometabolic health, aging, and longevity in ad libitum-fed mice* Cell Metab., 19 (2014), pp. 418-430

- S.J. Simpson, D. Raubenheime The Nature of Nutrition: a Unifying Framework from Animal Adaptation to Human Obesity Princeton Univ. Press, Princeton, NJ (2012)
- M. Ferguson, I. Rebrin, M.J. Forster, R.S. Sohal *Comparison of metabolic rate and oxidative stress between two different strains of mice with varying response to caloric restriction* Exp. Gerontol., 43 (2008), pp. 757-763
- R.N. Butler, R. Sprott, H. Warner, J. Bland, R. Feuers, M. Forster, H. Fillit, S.M. Harman, M. Hewitt, M. Hyman, K. Johnson, E. Kligman, G. McClearn, J. Nelson, A. Richardson, W. Sonntag, R. Weindruch, N. Wolf *Biomarkers of aging: from primitive organisms to humans* J. Gerontol. A Biol. Sci. Med. Sci., 59 (2004), pp. B560-B567
- M.E. Reff, E.L. Schneider *Biological Markers of Aging* U.S. Govt. Printing Office, Washington, DC (1982)
- R.L. Sprott *Biomarkers of aging* J. Gerontol. A Biol. Sci. Med. Sci., 54 (1999), pp. B464-B465
- R.L. Sprott *Development of animal models of aging at the National Institute on Aging* Neurobiol. Aging, 12 (1991), pp. 635-638
- N. Barzilai, G. Gupta *Revisiting the role of fat mass in the life extension induced by caloric restriction* J. Gerontol. A Biol. Sci. Med. Sci., 54 (1999), pp. B89-B96 (discussion B97-B98)
- D.E. Harrison, J.R. Archer, C.M. Astle *Effects of food restriction on aging: separation of food intake and adiposity* Proc. Natl. Acad. Sci. USA, 81 (1984), pp. 1835-1838
- P. Schrauwen, V. Schrauwen-Hinderling, J. Hoeks, M.K. Hesselink *Mitochondrial dysfunction and lipotoxicity* Biochim. Biophys. Acta, 1801

- N.L. Nadon *Exploiting the rodent model for studies on the pharmacology of lifespan extension* Aging Cell, 5 (2006), pp. 9-15
- A.J. Dirks, C. Leeuwenburgh *Caloric restriction in humans: potential pitfalls and health concerns* Mech. Ageing Dev., 127 (2006), pp. 1-7
- E.A. Moreira, M. Most, J. Howard, E. Ravussin *Dietary adherence to long-term controlled feeding in a calorie-restriction study in overweight men and women* Nutr. Clin. Pract., 26 (2011), pp. 309-315
- B.J. Merry *Molecular mechanisms linking calorie restriction and longevity*
- Int. J. Biochem. Cell Biol., 34 (2002), pp. 1340-1354
- Y. Li, M. Daniel, T.O. Tollefsbol *Epigenetic regulation of caloric restriction in aging* BMC Med., 9 (2011), p. 98
- S. Libert, L. Guarente *Metabolic and neuropsychiatric effects of calorie restriction and sirtuins* Annu. Rev. Physiol., 75 (2013), pp. 669-684
- R.S. Sohal, R. Weindruch *Oxidative stress, caloric restriction, and aging* Science, 273 (1996), pp. 59-63
- P.C. Withers, C.E. Cooper *Metabolic depression: a historical perspective* Prog. Mol. Subcell. Biol., 49 (2010), pp. 1-23
- Olshansky, S. J.; Hayflick, L; Carnes, B. A. (1 August 2002). "Position statement on human aging". The Journals of Gerontology Series A: Biological Sciences and Medical Sciences. **57** *(8):* B292–7.
- Warner H, Anderson J, Austad S; et al. (2005). "Science fact and the SENS agenda. What can we reasonably expect from ageing research?". EMBO Reports. **6** *(11):* 1006–8.

- López-Otín, C; Blasco, M. A.; Partridge, L; Serrano, M; Kroemer, G (2013). "The hallmarks of aging". Cell. **153** (6): 1194–1217.
- Halliwell B, Gutteridge JMC (2007). *Free Radicals in Biology and Medicine*. Oxford University Press, USA, ISBN 019856869X, ISBN 978-0198568698
- Holmes, G. E.; Bernstein, C; Bernstein, H (September 1992). "Oxidative and other DNA damages as the basis of aging: a review". Mutation Research/DNAging. **275** (3–6): 305–15.
- Verdaguer, E; Junyent, F; Folch, J; Beas-Zarate, C; Auladell, C; Pallàs, M; Camins, A (2012). "*Aging biology: a new frontier for drug discovery*". Expert Opin Drug Discov. **7** (3): 217–229.
- Rauser, C. L.; Mueller, L. D.; Rose, M. R. (2006). "The evolution of late life". Ageing Res Rev. **5** (1): 14–32.
- Stearns, S. C.; Ackermann, M; Doebeli, M; Kaiser, M (2000). "*Experimental evolution of aging, growth, and reproduction in fruitflies*". Proceedings of the National Academy of Sciences of the United States of America. **97** (7): 3309–3313.
- "Not your father's planarian: a classic model enters the era of functional genomics". Nat Rev Genet. **3** (3): 210–219.
- Martínez DE (May 1998). "*Mortality patterns suggest lack of senescence in hydra*". Experimental Gerontology. **33** (3): 217–25.
- Petralia, Ronald S.; Mattson, Mark P.; Yao, Pamela J. (2014). "Aging and longevity in the simplest animals and the quest for immortality". Ageing Res Rev. **16**: 66–82.
- Redman LM, Heilbronn LK, Martin CK, de Jonge L, Williamson DA, Delany JP, Ravussin E (2009). "*Metabolic and behavioral compensations in response to caloric restriction: implications for the*

- *maintenance of weight loss". PLOS ONE. 4 (2): e4377.*
- Holloszy JO; Fontana L (2007). "Caloric restriction in humans". Exp Gerontol. **42** (8): 709–12. doi:10.1016/j.exger.2007.03.009. PMC 2020845. PMID 17482403.
- Mattison JA, Roth GS, Beasley TM; et al. (2012). "Impact of caloric restriction on health and survival in rhesus monkeys from the NIA study". Nature. **489** (7415): 318–321.
- Spindler, Stephen R. (2010). "Biological Effects of Calorie Restriction: Implications for Modification of Human Aging". The Future of Aging. pp. 367–438.
- Bjelakovic, Goran; Nikolova, Dimitrinka; Lotte Gluud, Lise; Simonetti Rosa G.; Gluud Christian (2007). "Mortality in Randomized Trials of Antioxidant Supplements for Primary and Secondary Prevention, a Systematic Review and Meta-analysis". JAMA. **297** (8): 842–857.
- Fernández AF; Fraga MF (Jul 2011). "The effects of the dietary polyphenol resveratrol on human healthy aging and lifespan". Epigenetics. **6** (7): 870–4.
- Sattler FR (August 2013). "Growth hormone in the aging male". Best Pract. Res. Clin. Endocrinol. Metab. **27** (4): 541–55.
- Stambler, Ilia (2014). *A History of Life-Extensionism in the Twentieth Century. Longevity History.* ISBN 1500818577.
- Hughes, James (October 20, 2011). "Transhumanism". In Bainbridge, William. *Leadership in Science and Technology: A Reference Handbook.* Sage Publications. p. 587. ISBN 1452266522.

- Clevenger, Ty (Summer 2000). "Internet pharmacies: cyberspace versus the regulatory state". Journal of Law and Health. Archived from the original on 18 September 2009. Retrieved 17 July 2009.
- West, Michael D. (2003). *The Immortal Cell: One Scientist's Quest to Solve the Mystery of Human Aging.* Doubleday. ISBN 978-0-385-50928-2.
- Stolyarov, Gennady *(November 25, 2013). Death is Wrong (PDF). Rational Argumentator Press. ISBN 978-0615932040.*
- Istvan, Zoltan (October 2, 2014). "The Morality of Artificial Intelligence and the Three Laws of Transhumanism". Huffington Post.
- Arion McNicoll, Arion (3 October 2013). "How Google's Calico aims to fight aging and 'solve death'". CNN.
- "Google announces Calico, a new company focused on health and well-being". Google. September 18, 2013.
- Wolpert, Stuart. "UCLA biologists delay the aging process by 'remote control'". UCLA.edu.
- *Kass, Leon (1985). Toward a more natural science: biology and human affairs. New York City: Free Press. p. 316. ISBN 978-0-02-918340-3.*
- Harris J. (2007) *Enhancing Evolution: The ethical case for making better people.* Princeton University Press, New Jersey.
- Sutherland, John (9 May 2006). "The ideas interview: Nick Bostrom". The Guardian. London. Retrieved 17 July 2009.
- Bostrom, N (May 2005). "The fable of the dragon tyrant". Journal of Medical Ethics. **31** (5): 273–7.

- Sandel, Michael J. (2004), *"The Case against Perfection"*, The Atlantic Monthly, (April 2004), 51-62.
- Schloendorn, John (2006), *"Making the Case for Human Life-extension: Personal Arguments"*, Bioethics, 20 (4), 191-202.
- Singer, Peter (1991), *"Research into Aging: Should It Be Guided by the Interests of Present Individuals, Future Individuals, or the Species?"*, in Frederic C. Ludwig (ed.), Life Span Extension: Consequences and Open Questions (New York: Springer).
- Temkin, Larry (2011), "Is Living Longer Living Better?", in Julian Savulescu, Ruud ter Meulen, and Guy Kahane (eds.), *Enhancing Human Capacities* (Oxford: Wiley-Blackwell).
- Trotter, Griffin (2004), *"Why Bioethics Is Ill Equipped to Contribute to the Debate About Prolonging Lifespans"*, HEC Forum, 16 (3), 197-213.
- Velleman, J. David (1992), *"Against the Right to Die"*, The Journal of Medical Philosophy 17 (6), 665-81.
- Walker, Mark (2007), *"Superlongevity and Utilitarianism"*, Australasian Journal of Philosophy, 85 (4), 581-95.
- Weinstein, Neil D. (1980), *"Unrealistic Optimism About Future Life Events"*, Journal of Personality and Social Psychology, 39 (5), 806-20.

- Hillman CH, Erickson KI, Kramer AF (2008) *Be smart, exercise your heart: Exercise effects on brain and cognition.* Nat Rev Neurosci 9:58–65.
- van Praag H, Shubert T, Zhao C, Gage FH (2005) *Exercise enhances learning and hippocampal*

neurogenesis in aged mice. J Neurosci 25:8680–8685.
- Cotman CW, Berchtold NC(2002) Exercise: *A behavioral intervention to enhance brain health and plasticity.* Trends Neurosci 25:295–301.
- Creer DJ, Romberg C, Saksida LM, van Praag H, Bussey TJ(2010) Running enhances spatial pattern separation in mice. Proc Natl Acad Sci USA 107:2367–2372.
- Vaynman S, Ying Z, Gomez-Pinilla F(2004) *Hippocampal BDNF mediates the efficacy of exercise on synaptic plasticity and cognition.* Eur J Neurosci 20:2580–2590.
- Li Y, et al.(2008) TrkB regulates hippocampal neurogenesis and governs sensitivity to antidepressive treatment. Neuron 59:399–412.
- Colcombe SJ, et al.(2006) *Aerobic exercise training increases brain volume in aging humans.* J Gerontol A Biol Sci Med Sci 61:1166–1170.
- Colcombe SJ, et al.(2004) *Cardiovascular fitness, cortical plasticity, and aging.* Proc Natl Acad Sci USA 101:3316–3321.
- Rosano C, et al.(2010) *Psychomotor speed and functional brain MRI 2 years after completing a physical activity treatment.* J Gerontol A Biol Sci Med Sci 65:639–647.
- Erickson KI, et al.(2010) *Physical activity predicts gray matter volume in late adulthood: The Cardiovascular Health Study.* Neurology 75:1415–1422.
- Erickson KI, et al.(2009) Aerobic fitness is associated with hippocampal volume in elderly humans. Hippocampus 19:1030–1039.
- Honea RA, et al.(2009) *Cardiorespiratory fitness and preserved medial temporal lobe volume in*

Alzheimer's disease. Alzheimer Dis Assoc Disord 23:188–197.
- Pereira AC, et al.(2007) An in vivo correlate of exercise-induced neurogenesis in the
- Burdette JH, et al.(2010) *Using network science to evaluate exercise-associated brain changes in older adults.* Front Aging Neurosci 2:23.
- Moser MB, Moser EI, Forrest E, Andersen P, Morris RG(1995) *Spatial learning with a minislab in the dorsal hippocampus.* Proc Natl Acad Sci USA 92:9697–9701.
- Raji CA, Lopez OL, Kuller LH, Carmichael OT, Becker JT(2009) *Age, Alzheimer disease, and brain structure.* Neurology 73:1899–1905.
- Hackert VH, et al.(2002) *Hippocampal head size associated with verbal memory performance in nondemented elderly.* Neuroimage 17:1365–1372.
- Neeper SA, Gómez-Pinilla F, Choi J, Cotman C(1995) *Exercise and brain neurotrophins.* Nature 373:109.
- Homes MM, Galea LA, Mistlberger RE, Kempermann G(2004) *Adult hippocampal neurogenesis and voluntary running activity: Circadian and dose-dependent effects.* J Neurosci Res 76:216–222.
- Erickson KI, et al.(2010) *Brain-derived neurotrophic factor is associated with age-related decline in hippocampal volume.* J Neurosci 30:5368–5375.
- Kramer AF, et al.(1999) Ageing, fitness and neurocognitive function. Nature 400:418–419.
- Colcombe SJ, Kramer AF(2003) *Fitness effects on the cognitive function of older adults: A meta-analytic study.* Psychol Sci 14:125–130.
- Smith PJ, et al.(2010) *Aerobic exercise and neurocognitive performance: A meta-analytic*

- *review of randomized controlled trials.* Psychosom Med 72:239-252.
- Rasmussen P, et al.(2009) *Evidence for a release of brain-derived neurotrophic factor from the brain during exercise.* Exp Physiol 94:1062-1069.
- Zoladz J, et al.(2008) *Endurance training increases plasma brain-derived neurotrophic factor concentration in young healthy men.* J Physiol Pharmacol 59(Suppl 7):119-132.
- Lee R, Kermani P, Teng KK, Hempstead BL2001) *Regulation of cell survival by secreted proneurotrophins.* Science 294:1945-1948.
- Pencea V, Bingaman KD, Wiegand SJ, Luskin MB(2001) *Infusion of brain-derived neurotrophic factor into the lateral ventricle of the adult rat leads to new neurons in the parenchyma of the striatum, septum, thalamus, and hypothalamus.* J Neurosci 21:6706-6717.
- Figurov A, Pozzo-Miller LD, Olafsson P, Wang T, Lu B(1996) *Regulation of synaptic responses to high-frequency stimulation and LTP by neurotrophins in the hippocampus.* Nature 381:706-709.
- Black JE, Isaacs KR, Anderson BJ, Alcantara AA, Greenough WT(1990) *Learning causes synaptogenesis, whereas motor activity causes angiogenesis, in cerebellar cortex of adult rats.* Proc Natl Acad Sci USA 87:5568-5572.
- Redila VA, Christie BR(2006) *Exercise-induced changes in dendritic structure and complexity in the adult hippocampal dentate gyrus.* Neuroscience 137:1299-1307.
- Strath SJ, et al.(2000) *Evaluation of heart rate as a method for assessing moderate intensity physical*

activity. Med Sci Sports Exerc 32((9 Suppl)) S465–S470.
- Heo S, et al.(2010) *Resting hippocampal blood flow, spatial memory and aging.* Brain Res 1315:119–127.

About the Author

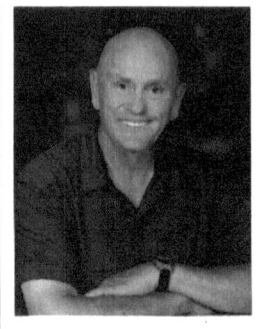

Mark Roberts-Seymour, B.A.Sc., P.Eng., CD, ACG, OFS is a Canadian Professional Forensic Engineer, a recognised stoneworks conservator, Chartered Demographer, non-fiction author, lay-brother and comparative theologian, professional public speaker (Toastmaster Advanced Communicator Gold), technical paper referee, statistical assessor, and editor.

Over succeeding years his publications have included:

- *Generationiism: Is It Significant*
- *Canadian Sub-Urban Self-Sufficiency*
- *Christian Transmigration*
- *Old, Unemployed and Pissed: Late Career Canadians Coping with Long-term Unemployment*
- *Seniors Life Extension*

- *Restructuring a Broken Canadian Economic-Democracy*
- *Three Proto-Christian Orthodoxies, The Gospel of Paul, Alexandrian Orthodoxy and Proto-Christian Gnosticism: A Comparison*
- *Clinical Happiness: Measurement, Measures, Goals and Habit Conditioning*
- *Anglicanism: From Henry to Henrietta*
- *Cyborg:* Smartphone Reliance, AI and Transhumanism
- *An Afterlife:* Who Cares! Quotations on an After-life with Biographical notes
- *Conservation of Heritage Cemeteries,*
- *Green Revolutions – Will they be Enough,*
- *Suburban and Ex-Urban Self Sufficiency,*
- *Life Extension for Seniors Book 1: Expectations, Ageing Inhibition, Nutrition, Brain 'Wiring', Habits, Exercise and Ethics*
- *The Working Poor: Who are Poor and What Can Be Done: A Central British Columbia Case Study*
- *Life Extension for Seniors Book 2: Methods, Research, Supplementation, Health and Life-Prolonging Strategies*
- *Abrahamic Gnosticism is not Scary,*
- *Proofs of God – Philosophy of Religion and Science Converge,*
- *Anglicanism – From Henry to Henrietta,*
- *Happiness: Biochemistry, Goals and Habituation,*
- *The Parable of the Prodigal Son - Death, Rebirth, Recognition and Reconciliation,*
- *Nutrition for Older Workers,*

Seniors Life Extension

- *Nutrient Supplements for the Older Worker*,
- *Canadian Systems: Changing our Economic-Democracy*,
- *Gnosticism as Revelation: from St. Paul to C.G. Jung*,
- *Sabotage, Wealth and New Classes*,
- *Christian Metempsychosis: Elijah and John the Baptist*,
- *Sanctification – It's for Everyone!*,
- *The Gospel of Paul, Christian Gnosticism and Alexandrian Orthodoxy – A Comparison*,
- *An Afterlife, Who Cares!* **Quotations from 231 sources**
- *Renovating the Canadian Economic-Democratic System*,
- *To Coin a Phrase or Not to Coin a Phrase: Cliches, Metaphors and Euphemisms in Use*,
- *Canadian Systems: Changing our Economic-Democracy*,
- *It Can't Happen Here: Future Mechanisation, Despair and Suicide*

To access further information on these books [or for purchase], links to the Distributor Amazon.com are indicated in the list preceding.

Mark acted for more thirty years as a Registered Professional Engineer (P.Eng., PE, ing.), technical author and editor for: The Government of BC (Lands Forests and Water Resources), BH Levelton and Associates, Warnock Hersey Professional Services, Heritage Technologies

Press, RM Hardy and Associates, G.W. Spratt Limited and others. Mark also owned and managed a private Materials Engineering firm for an additional ten years (Roberts Seymour and Associates Limited).

He remains active in several service, political and social justice organisations as well as maintaining his professional standings. He is married, the father of four adult children and many grandchildren, and calls Vernon, British Columbia, Canada his home. Mark Roberts-Seymour can be reached directly by email at merscanada@gmail.com and by telephone at (250) 309-8350. For keynote speaking and seminar leadership contact (778) 721-5683.

www.ingramcontent.com/pod-product-compliance
Lightning Source LLC
Chambersburg PA
CBHW031615210526
45464CB00004B/1593